Psycho-Socio-Physical Dimensions of Adolescent Health Management:

Emerging Research and Opportunities

Sapna Nanda
Panjab University, India

A volume in the Advances in Human Services and Public Health (AHSPH) Book Series

IGI Global
DISSEMINATOR OF KNOWLEDGE

Published in the United States of America by
IGI Global
Medical Information Science Reference (an imprint of IGI Global)
701 E. Chocolate Avenue
Hershey PA, USA 17033
Tel: 717-533-8845
Fax: 717-533-8661
E-mail: cust@igi-global.com
Web site: http://www.igi-global.com

Library of Congress Cataloging-in-Publication Data

Names: Nanda, Sapna, 1964- author.
Title: Psycho-socio-physical dimensions of adolescent health management : emerging research and opportunities / by Sapna Nanda.
Description: Hershey, PA : Medical Information Science Reference, [2019] | Includes bibliographical references.
Identifiers: LCCN 2018025682| ISBN 9781522573845 (hardcover) | ISBN 9781522573852 (ebook)
Subjects: | MESH: Adolescent Health
Classification: LCC RJ503 | NLM WS 460 | DDC 616.8900835--dc23 LC record available at https://lccn.loc.gov/2018025682

This book is published in the IGI Global book series Advances in Human Services and Public Health (AHSPH) (ISSN: 2475-6571; eISSN: 2475-658X)

British Cataloguing in Publication Data
A Cataloguing in Publication record for this book is available from the British Library.

All work contributed to this book is new, previously-unpublished material.
The views expressed in this book are those of the authors, but not necessarily of the publisher.

For electronic access to this publication, please contact: eresources@igi-global.com.

Advances in Human Services and Public Health (AHSPH) Book Series

ISSN:2475-6571
EISSN:2475-658X

Editor-in-Chief: Jennifer Martin, RMIT University, Australia

MISSION

The well-being of the general public should be a primary concern for any modern civilization. Ongoing research in the field of human services and public healthcare is necessary to evaluate, manage, and respond to the health and social needs of the global population.

The **Advances in Human Services and Public Health (AHSPH)** book series aims to publish high-quality reference publications focused on the latest methodologies, tools, issues, and strategies for managing the health and social welfare of the public. The AHSPH book series will be especially relevant for healthcare professionals, policy makers, government officials, and students seeking the latest research in this field.

COVERAGE

- Public Funding
- Assistance Programs
- Domestic Violence
- Healthcare Reform
- Medicare and Medicaid
- Social Welfare Policy
- Social Work
- Access to Healthcare Services
- Public Welfare
- Health policy

IGI Global is currently accepting manuscripts for publication within this series. To submit a proposal for a volume in this series, please contact our Acquisition Editors at Acquisitions@igi-global.com or visit: http://www.igi-global.com/publish/.

The Advances in Human Services and Public Health (AHSPH) Book Series (ISSN 2475-6571) is published by IGI Global, 701 E. Chocolate Avenue, Hershey, PA 17033-1240, USA, www.igi-global.com. This series is composed of titles available for purchase individually; each title is edited to be contextually exclusive from any other title within the series. For pricing and ordering information please visit http://www.igi-global.com/book-series/advances-human-services-public-health/102256. Postmaster: Send all address changes to above address.

Titles in this Series

For a list of additional titles in this series, please visit:
https://www.igi-global.com/book-series/advances-human-services-public-health/102256

Socio-Cultural Influences on Teenage Pregnancy and Contemporary Prevention Measures
Devi Akella (Albany State Universty, USA)
Information Science Reference • ©2019 • 349pp • H/C (ISBN: 9781522561088) • US $195.00

Nutraceutical and Functional Foods in Disease Prevention
Raj K. Keservani (Chhatrapati Shahu Ji Maharaj Group of Institutions, India) Anil K. Sharma (Delhi Institute of Pharmaceutical Sciences and Research, India) and Rajesh K. Kesharwani (Nims University Rajasthan, India)
Medical Information Science Reference • ©2019 • 569pp • H/C (ISBN: 9781522532675) • US $215.00

Ethical Issues in Social Work Practice
Antonio Sandu (Ştefan cel Mare University of Suceava, Romania) and Ana Frunza (LUMEN Research Center in Social and Humanistic Sciences, Romania)
Information Science Reference • ©2018 • 328pp • H/C (ISBN: 9781522530909) • US $195.00

Global Perspectives on Human Migration, Asylum, and Security
Christina M. Akrivopoulou (Hellenic Open University, Greece)
Information Science Reference • ©2018 • 268pp • H/C (ISBN: 9781522528173) • US $185.00

Nutraceuticals and Innovative Food Products for Healthy Living and Preventive Care
Amit Verma (SDAU, India) Kajal Srivastava (GBPUAT, India) Shivom Singh (ITM University, India) and Hukum Singh (Forest Research Institute, India)
Medical Information Science Reference • ©2018 • 462pp • H/C (ISBN: 9781522529705) • US $245.00

Health Information Systems and the Advancement of Medical Practice in Developing...
Kgomotso H. Moahi (University of Botswana, Botswana) Kelvin Joseph Bwalya (University of Johannesburg, South Africa) and Peter Mazebe II Sebina (University of Botswana, Botswana)
Medical Information Science Reference • ©2017 • 350pp • H/C (ISBN: 9781522522621) • US $200.00

Examining the Role of Environmental Change on Emerging Infectious Diseases and...
Maha Bouzid (University of East Anglia, UK)
Information Science Reference • ©2017 • 327pp • H/C (ISBN: 9781522505532) • US $200.00

For an entire list of titles in this series, please visit:
https://www.igi-global.com/book-series/advances-human-services-public-health/102256

IGI Global
DISSEMINATOR OF KNOWLEDGE

701 East Chocolate Avenue, Hershey, PA 17033, USA
Tel: 717-533-8845 x100 • Fax: 717-533-8661
E-Mail: cust@igi-global.com • www.igi-global.com

Table of Contents

Foreword vii

Preface x

Acknowledgment xix

Introduction xxi

Chapter 1
Introduction 1

Chapter 2
Physical Health 22

Chapter 3
Psycho-Social Health 66

Chapter 4
Sexual and Reproductive Health 101

Chapter 5
Adolescent Health Management 118

Chapter 6
Summary and Conclusion 160

Glossary clxx

Related Readings 178

About the Author 199

Index 200

Foreword

According to the World Health Organization (1995), "One of the most important commitments a country can make for its future economic, social and political progress and stability is to address the health and developmental needs of its adolescents." The health of adolescents can be defined by traditional measures such as mortality rates, incidence of disease and prevalence of chronic disease conditions. A more complex and complete picture of adolescent health status, however, also encompasses the prevalence of various leading adolescent behaviors and health outcomes as well as health indicators that may adversely affect their health status in adulthood.

Adolescence is a critical transitional period that includes the biological changes of puberty and developmental tasks such as normative exploration and learning to be independent. Adolescents who have reached adulthood also face significant social and economic challenges with few organizational supports at a time when they are expected to take on adult responsibilities and obligations.

Adolescents and young adults make up about 28% of the total India's population. Although adolescence and young adulthood are comparatively healthier times of life, some important health and social problems either start or peak during these years. The behavioral patterns established during these developmental periods help determine young people's current health status and their risk for developing chronic diseases during adulthood.

Young people's vulnerability to risky or unwanted sex and other unhealthy behaviors is associated with a host of individual, familial and community factors that influence their behavior and that are closely related to their economic and educational opportunities. Good health and other physical, moral and intellectual developmental outcomes are often mutually reinforcing. For example, healthy children do better in academics in schools. Conversely, having more years of schooling provides essential information and skills that are linked to more protective, healthy and less risky behaviors.

Poverty and inadequate health care systems further compound adolescent's vulnerability to diseases and premature deaths. At the same time, poor health exacerbates poverty by disrupting and cutting short school opportunities, by weakening or killing young people in the prime of their working lives or by placing heavy financial and social burdens on their families.

Improving the health status of adolescents and young adults is complex and difficult, more so than for other age groups. As compared to children, adolescents are less protected by their families and communities and less amenable to simple solutions to their health problems, many of which are behaviour-based. Compared to adults, adolescents know less about how to stay healthy and have fewer resources to prevent or treat their health problems. In contrast, their behaviors are less firmly entrenched and they are often involved in institutional activities, such as schools, training programs etc. where programs with high coverage can be sustained.

Research from various sources as well as the experiences of adolescents and health care providers, health organizations and research centers suggest the importance of designing health services that can attract and engage adolescents, create opportunities to discuss sensitive health and behavioural issues and offer high-quality care as well as guidance for both health promotion and disease prevention. Programs will have to seek multi-sectoral solutions that link health sector interventions with other types of interventions delivered through other sectors, either at the program level or at the policy level.

With so many programs for adolescents available in India, the services have not reached the target group adequately because resources like materials, money and man power are limited. There is no direct access, space for privacy and ideal timings for the target population. Service providers are not given proper training. For the health care providers, it is usually an extra burden because no man power has been allotted separately for adolescent health services. Adolescents have little knowledge about the need of health services. They are scared of revealing personal issues to another person and getting examined by opposite sex health worker. So they themselves act as major obstacle for the services to reach them.

If the nations invest in health, education and job creation for adolescents, the resulting economic gains will improve their overall quality of life. Life skill education, particularly for adolescent girls, is strongly related to their reproductive behavior. In most countries, girls who are educated are more likely to delay marriage and childbearing, whereas girls with less education are more likely to become mothers as adolescents. Unfortunately, the causal relationships involved are not clear.

The difficulty in attributing improvements in health outcomes among adolescents to interventions delivered in multiple settings or sectors reflects the challenges involved. Programs aimed at young people are relatively new and untested. Nevertheless, accumulated experience, backed by an increasing body of research, has created international consensus around a multi-intervention approach.

To deal with such dilemmas, the empowerment of adolescents is a major concern of parents, teachers and the government. There are various opinions about the developmental needs of adolescents and the strategies to be followed for the same. Life skills-based education is one of the major strategies adopted across the world for empowerment of adolescents.

The focus of this manuscript is on emerging research and opportunities in the management of psych-socio-physical health of adolescents which has been presented very vividly so as to sensitize various stakeholders to the challenges and plan strategies of the effective management of adolescent health.

R. Puri
Panjab University, India

REFERENCES

World Health Organization, United Nations Population Fund, and United Nations Children's Fund. (1995). *Action for Adolescent Health: Towards a Common Agenda: Recommendations from a Joint Study Group*. Retrieved from http://www.who.int/child_adolescent_health/documents/frh_adh_97_9/en/index.html

Preface

The promotion of adolescent health has gained priority in recent years throughout the world for a number of varied reasons. Among those varied reasons, one is the changing environment in which adolescents live and the impact that the environment has on their behavior, which in turn, has implications for their health and wellbeing both in the short term as well as in the long term. The changing nature of adolescent health problems calls for new responses from the health sector to promote and protect adolescent health and, in turn, health and well being of the future generations.

According to a UN report (United Nations, 2014), youth in the age group of 10-24 years constitute more than 28% of total India's population. This population is an enormous potential resource for social as well as economic development of the country like India. The health status, needs and aspirations of this growing population determine the future progress of the nation. It is beyond doubt that nations with large youth population could see their economies soar, provided they invest heavily in health and education of this young population and protect their human rights.

The Committee on the rights of children and adolescents has issued guidelines on State's obligations to recognize the special health and developmental needs as well as rights of adolescents and young people. This has been further envisaged in WHO report in 2014 titled "Health for the world's adolescents".

The importance of investing in youth has also been recognized in India's Constitution. One of the Directive Principles of State Policy states that "It is imperative that children are given opportunities and facilities to develop in a healthy manner and in conditions of freedom and dignity and that childhood and youth are protected against exploitation and against moral and material abandonment" (Constitution of India, n.d.).

Youth is considered as a powerful segment of the society which decides the workforce and its efficiency to fulfill the sustainable development of any country. Empowering youth through effective and innovative programs leads to increase in productivity, adaptation of technology, up-graded process and speedy economic growth.

Adolescence, the critical phase of life, is a period of major physical, physiological, psychological and behavioural changes with changing patterns of social interactions and relationships. It is the window of opportunities that set the stage for a healthy and productive adulthood and to reduce the likelihood of health problems in later years. Adolescence (10-19 years) is, thus, the most susceptible and important phase in an individual's life and is a transitional phase between childhood and adulthood when the child moves from dependency to autonomy.

The needs and concerns of adolescents during this period of life are manifold. During this phase of life, they find themselves in utter confusion and many at times fall into crisis and troubles due to lack of proper guidance and support. Adolescents are vary of asking their parents, teachers or significant others for clarification of their doubts which affect them physically, psychologically or socially.

The physical concerns of adolescents like body growth and functions during puberty, body image and size, health and hygiene especially personal hygiene, idolizing styles of famous personalities, concern about their skin, colour, complexion, nutrition and food habits, fashion, reproductive health, sex and sexuality, responsible sexual behavior accompanying physical changes as well as coping disabilities warrant immediate attention. A myriad of biological changes occurring during puberty include increase in height and weight, completion of skeletal growth accompanied by an increase in skeletal mass, sexual maturation and changes in body composition. The succession of these events during puberty is generally consistent among the adolescents but is often influenced by age of onset of menarche, gender, duration etc. along with the individual variations in their growth pattern.

The psychological concerns of adolescents are even more delicate and sensitive and also very difficult to handle. The physical and physiological changes during puberty are accompanied by significant stress on young people and those around them while influencing and affecting their relationships with peers and adults. It is also an age of impulsivity accompanied by vulnerability, influenced by peer groups and media that often result in changes in their perception and practices and are usually characterized by decision making skills/abilities along with the acquisition of new emotional, cognitive and social skills. Identity formation and identity crisis, self-confidence and self-dissonance, self-esteem and self-acceptance, career aspirations and career guidance, lack of interest in academics, over indulgence in internet and social media, peer influence and peer pressure, infatuation and attraction towards opposite sex, impulsive and risky behaviour, tendency to self-harm and emotional outbursts etc. are quite common among the adolescents and they find it difficult to handle the pressure emanating from all such issues.

It is not only about physical or psychological issues that affect the adolescents in their day-to-day life. There is a whole spectrum of social concerns also which require immediate attention. Parental care and support, parent-child conflicts, erosion of values, including disrespect to elders, especially teachers, interpersonal relationships and peer influence, influence of media especially social media, familial and societal pressures etc. affect the social life of adolescents.

Available evidences indicate that adolescents and youth are also prone to a number of health impacting conditions due to personal choices, environmental influences and lifestyle changes, including both communicable and non-communicable disorders and injuries. Other health impacting conditions include substance use disorders (tobacco, alcohol and others), road traffic injuries (RTI's), suicides (completed or attempted), sexually transmitted infections (STI's), including Human Immunodeficiency Virus (HIV) infection, teen and unplanned pregnancies, homelessness, violence and several others. In all countries, whether developing, transitional or developed, disabilities and acute or chronic illnesses are often induced or compounded by economic hardship, unemployment, sanctions, restrictions, poverty or poorly or unevenly distributed wealth at both individual and country level.

Besides, certain groups of adolescents have particularly high rates of co-morbidities, defined as the simultaneous occurrence of two or more diseases, health conditions or risky behaviors. These adolescents are particularly vulnerable to high rates of morbidity and mortality. Moreover, specific groups of adolescents such as those who are below poverty line; in the foster care system; homeless; in families that have recently immigrated or in the juvenile justice system etc. may have still higher rates of chronic health problems and may even engage in more risky behavior as compared to the overall adolescent population.

Although majority of the adolescents are apparently healthy, but they are indulged in practicing unhealthy behaviors that ultimately result in much death and disability. This is an immense public health issue which needs the attention of the stakeholders concerned with adolescent health care. Therefore, focusing attention both on diseases experienced during adolescence and on risk factors with their roots in adolescence and growing into adulthood makes sense.

Concerted efforts on adolescent health care should focus on prevention because so much of the disease burden among adolescents is preventable. Since prevention is particularly a cost-effective strategy in relation to adolescent health, given the long duration over which the benefits will be reaped and adolescents' greater openness and flexibility to change as compared to adults. Since they are in developmental transition, adolescents and young adults (AYA's) are particularly sensitive to the influences from their social environment. Their parents, families, peer groups, schools and neighborhoods can either support or threaten young people's health and well-being. Societal policies and cues, such as structural racism and media messages, can also do the same.

However, older adolescents and young adults, including those with chronic health conditions, may face challenges as they transit from the child to the adult health care system, such as changes in their insurance coverage and legal status as well as the decreased attention to their developmental and behavioral needs. Bolstering the positive development of young people facilitates their adoption of healthy behaviors and helps ensure a healthy and productive adult population.

Existing adolescent health care programs focus on rendering services like nutrition education, dietary and nutrient supplementation, health education for sexual and reproductive health care, immunization, anemia and goiter control measures, vocational guidance and career counseling and so on. These adolescent health care programs in India are fragmentary at present and there is no comprehensive program addressing all the developmental needs of adolescents. Access and availability of health care services are also severely limited. Lack of accurate information, absence of proper guidance, parent's ignorance, lack of skills and insufficient services from health care delivery system are some of the major barriers in achieving the objective of healthy development of adolescents.

In such a scenario, there is an urgent need to provide today's adolescents and youth with new set of ways and systems to deal with the changing demands and challenges of life. Since the 'individual' rather than the 'system' is recognized as the basic unit of the society, it is essential that the adolescents be helped to develop various skills inherently to handle a wide variety of choices, changes and the stressors.

One best practice model for contributing to the healthy development of adolescents and youth is a life skills approach. A key aspect of human development - as important to basic survival as intellect - is the acquisition of socio-cognitive and emotional coping skills. This has been shown to have an impact on healthy behaviour of adolescents.

For more than a decade, researches on interventions that address these specific socio-cognitive and emotional coping skill areas have shown their effectiveness in promoting desirable behaviors such as sociability, improved communication, effective decision making and conflict resolution as well as preventing negative or high-risk behaviors such as use of tobacco, alcohol and other drugs, unsafe sex and violence. The family life and life skills education intervention is a good support system for adolescents at the community level.

To achieve the objective of wholesome adolescent health, there is an urgent need to have a multidimensional approach covering all aspects of adolescent health problems with special emphasis on physical, reproductive and mental health, behaviour change communication towards healthy lifestyle and positive social environment to acquire life skills.

Interventions on adolescent health care should focus on providing psychological and mental health services and behaviour change communication towards leading a healthy lifestyle, restricting advertisement related to junk food products, awareness generation about reproductive and sexual health, educating parents to prevent early marriage, teenage pregnancy and to counsel their children on nutrition and reproductive health. Universal coverage of adolescent friendly clinics is highly recommended. To be cost effective, all health care services addressing the adolescent's needs should come under single program.

Adolescent friendly clinics need to be widely established throughout the country and should achieve universal coverage. Screening of adolescent on regular basis could be an effective tool to detect and control the existing diseases and to avoid the occurrence of any new disease. Empower and involve adolescents in decision making that affects them and facilitates them with every opportunity for developing into a successful adult. Offering such opportunities to the growing adolescents gives them a chance to build a safe, happy, healthy and productive nation in the future.

Several alternative service approaches improve the health care system for adolescents to make services more accessible, acceptable, appropriate, effective and equitable. Such alternative service approaches are particularly important to support healthy development for those adolescents who are particularly more vulnerable to poor health or unhealthful habits and risky behaviors because of their demographic characteristics or other circumstances. However, limited evidence is available on health outcomes associated with alternative service approaches. Therefore, there is a need to identify areas of concern in which research could yield knowledge that would support qualitative improvement in the organization and delivery of health care services for adolescents.

There is a strongly felt need for public health community program to identify, prepare, integrate and implement activities that would help to promote health and healthy lifestyles of young people and establish mechanisms for delivery of population-based interventions along with measuring its impact. There is also a need to generate good quality and robust population data that can drive policies and programs. Strategic investments in health, nutrition, education, employment and welfare are critical for healthy growth of young people and these programs need to be monitored and evaluated for their efficacy and effectiveness using public health approaches.

ORGANIZATION OF THE BOOK

This book is organized into six chapters. A brief description of each of the chapter follows:

Chapter 1 introduces the readers to the most precious human resource i.e. adolescents who are the future of the nation, thus forming a major demographic and economic force. This phase of life is a window period of opportunities that sets the stage for healthy and productive adulthood. It highlights the importance of young people's health because of health impacting behaviours and conditions which affect their current health as well as health of future generations. This chapter gives an overview of global scenario as well as the problem status in India which calls for a strong need for intervention strategies that help to promote health and healthy lifestyles of this young population and establish mechanisms for their organization and delivery along with impact assessment that will assure these adolescents grow into healthy women, knowledgeable about themselves and their future goals and responsibilities, aware of the world around them, its opportunities and challenges and be able to be self-respecting and independent adults within the society.

Chapter 2 deals with the physical growth pattern of adolescents assessed through their nutritional health status, anthropometric measurements/ indices, catch-up growth, clinical manifestation of health and nutritional status, hematological profile, incidence of under-nutrition, overweight and obesity in the Indian scenario as well as in other parts of the world. It also reveals the impact of dietary and nutrient supplementation on their physical health through catch up growth. The findings of authors research on physical growth parameters of adolescents have been reviewed in the light of contemporary researches thereby focusing on challenges and opportunities for this group of population.

Chapter 3 focuses on psycho-social health of adolescents by highlighting on achieving identity as a key task of adolescence with a focus on psycho-social needs, challenges, psycho-social dysfunction, common mental disorders as well as the strategies to improve mental health status of adolescents as the adolescents are exposed to a number of risk factors like increased sexual desire and no outlet, peer pressure, aggression, victimization, bullying besides an addiction to alcohol and drugs, use of tobacco and other substance abuse, violence and injuries, depression, suicide thoughts etc. The review in this chapter is expected to bring out the hidden and neglected public health issues which could help to increase the attention of health planners and programmers to develop sufficient adolescent mental health programs.

Chapter 4 deals with sexual and reproductive health of adolescents, especially early pregnancy and childbirth, HIV/AIDS and other infectious diseases, maternal mortality and morbidity, need of exercise and nutrition to deal with such issues. The chapter also discusses the rights of adolescents to survive, grow and develop are enshrined in International legal documents. It highlights the obligations to recognize the special health and developmental needs and rights of adolescents and young people. In response, WHO carries out a wide range of functions to improve the health of young people including production of evidence-based guidelines to support health services in other sectors; making recommendations to governments on adolescent health and the provision of high quality age-appropriate health services for adolescents; documenting progress in adolescent health and development and also raising awareness on health issues of young people among the general public and other interested stakeholders.

Chapter 5 aims at management of adolescent health by emphasizing on the need of life skills for adolescents so as to enable them to develop the abilities for adaptive and positive behavior to deal effectively with the demands and challenges of everyday life and also explaining core life skills as prescribed by World Health Organization (WHO). This necessitates the need for more pragmatic and action-oriented approach for incorporating life skills education in the curriculum of primary and secondary school levels to inculcate these healthy skills to shape and steer child's thought process in the desired direction. More emphasis needs to be laid on all aspects of life skills realizing their importance in helping youth to be equipped with better coping skills. Since more and more non- government organizations have taken the initiative by considering these life skills as a potent weapon to empower the youngsters in these challenging times, their efforts must be strengthened by governmental initiatives in such programs.

Chapter 6 summarizes on the healthy development of adolescents by highlighting various dimensions of adolescent health and related issues which depends on several interactive and complex factors like socio-economic and environmental factors in which they are born and brought up, the interpersonal relationships they develop with their peers and other adults around them, values of the community in which they live and the opportunities they have for their education and employment. It also emphasizes on the need and importance of life skill education for adolescents so as to enable them to develop psycho-social competencies and inter-personal skills which help them to make informed decisions, communicate effectively and develop coping and self-management skills to lead a healthy and productive life.

However, exclusive data pertaining to the adolescent health issues in Indian scenario is not available as compared to other developing and developed countries. Nation and state-wise detailed investigations and reporting on adolescent's health issues is the need of the hour. This will help to create better awareness among the planners, policy makers as well as other stakeholders about the importance of strengthening adolescent health services under a single agency in order to meet their felt needs. Hence, youth should be properly nurtured and promoted through entrepreneurship activities and imparted employability skills. For that, both central and state governments have implemented many programs and schemes. Moreover, the policy makers should take proper mechanism to empower the youth in society-physically, economically and also politically.

The present manuscript is an attempt in this direction in order to sensitize the adolescents, parents, health care professionals, researchers and scholars as well as other stakeholders and the general public as well so as to understand the health needs of adolescents, strategize various health care programs, assess the impact of various health care approaches in modifying the health and behavior of adolescents and how life skills education intervention facilitates them to lead a healthy and positive life so as to enable them to discharge their duties as the productive and contributing members of the society.

Sapna Nanda
Panjab University, India

REFERENCES

Constitution of India. (n.d.). Directive Principles of State Policy, India (Part IV) (Articles 39-43) Para 39 (f). *The Constitution of India*. Retrieved from https://www.mea.gov.in/Images/pdf1/Part4.pdf

United Nations. (2014). *India has world's largest youth population.* United Nations Report. Retrieved from https://www.thehindu.com/todays-paper/tp-in-school/india-has-worlds-largest-youth-population-un-report/article6612615.ece

World Health Organization. (2014). *Health for the World's Adolescents: Disability Adjusted Life Years: Combining Mortality and Morbidity*. Available from: http://public.tableausoftware.com/profile/digitalteam#!/vizhome/shared/FPXZ7PPMR

Acknowledgment

It gives me immense pleasure in expressing gratitude to everyone who has lent me an unconditional support in the preparation of this manuscript.

I express my profound sense of reverence to my mentor Dr. (Mrs.) R. Puri, Professor Emeritus, Foods & Nutrition and Associate Dean (Ret.), College Development Council, Panjab University, Chandigarh for her scholarly inspiration, professional guidance and erudition throughout the course of my doctoral research work. Working under her guidance had been a rich and valuable learning and rewarding experience. Besides her professional inputs, her love, affection and blessings have sharpened my personality.

I acknowledge the contributions of all researchers who have been working in the area of adolescent health and their findings have enriched my knowledge and made my research meaningful and relevant in the light of contemporary researches.

I shall be failing in my duty if I do not express my heartfelt gratitude to the team of IGI Global Publishing of United States of America for their faith in my abilities that has been a steering force for initiating this project. I immensely appreciate the unconditional support of Ms. Jordan Tepper, my development editor for providing me the best technical assistance, intrinsic motivation, immediate feedback and reinforcement from time to time for successful accomplishment of this project.

I deeply acknowledge the contributions of my family and friends who have always been a source of inspiration and constructive suggestions that helped in improving the quality of this manuscript. I am deeply indebted to my husband and children for supporting me with their utmost patience and elevating my spirits for completion of this assignment.

Last but not the least, I must acknowledge and thank Almighty God for His blessings, directing and guiding me for this task. I could never have accomplished this task without faith in His powers.

Sapna Nanda
Panjab University, India

Introduction

Adolescence, the second decade of life, is a period of transition from childhood to adulthood marked by rapid changes, which are physical, social and psychological in nature. Of the 12 million girls born in India every year, 1.5 million girls die before the age of one and one out of every four does not live to celebrate her fifteenth birthday due to gender discrimination and gross neglect. This can be linked to neglect of females as infants, as children, as adolescents and as mothers. Accidents, violence and suicides are the three most common causes of death among adolescents. Impaired mental and emotional health is a precursor or consequence of many health-risk behaviours such as physical, sexual or emotional abuse; reckless driving or excessive risk taking; extreme eating habits and excessive influence of advertisement or other forms of media. Other adolescent behaviour and attitudes are also integrally linked to adolescent mental health. These dilemmas arise out of everyday issues like peer influence, dating identity, emerging sexuality, independence, separation, identity crises, anxiety and responsibility as well as more serious ones like violent behavior, experimental sex, teenage suicides and other health related disorders. For the health management of adolescents, 'psychological and interpersonal skills' need to be acquired to help them to communicate better, to make more informed and balanced decisions, to avoid risky situations and to cope with stress as these life skills shape attitudes and ultimately lead to pro-social behaviour and productive life styles. 'Life skills' are, thus, the abilities for adaptive and positive behaviour that enable adolescents to deal effectively with the demands and challenges of everyday life.

Chapter 1
Introduction

ABSTRACT

Adolescence, the second decade of life, is a period of transition from childhood to adulthood marked by rapid changes, which are physical, social, and psychological in nature. Of the 12 million girls born in India every year, 1.5 million girls die before the age of one and one out of every four does not live to celebrate her fifteenth birthday due to gender discrimination and gross neglect. This can be linked to neglect of females as infants, as children, as adolescents, and as mothers. Impaired mental and emotional health is a precursor or consequence of many health-risk behaviors such as physical, sexual, social, or emotional abuse. These dilemmas arise out of everyday issues like peer influence, dating identity, emerging sexuality, independence, separation, identity crises, anxiety, and responsibility as well as more serious ones like violent behavior, experimental sex, teenage suicides, and other health-related disorders.

KEY FACTS

- India is one of the largest demographic countries in this world, with 22.1 percent of youth available in the country (Paramasivan & Kumaresan, 2016).
- About 34 percent of India's Gross National Income (GNI) is contributed by the youth, aged 15-29 years (Paramasivan & Kumaresan, 2016).

DOI: 10.4018/978-1-5225-7384-5.ch001

- Worldwide, there are more than 1.2 billion adolescents who indicate that roughly one in every six persons is an adolescent (UNICEF, 2012).
- In India, about 2 percent of total population is adolescent which constitutes about 243 million adolescents (Government of India, 2014).

INTRODUCTION

Youth constitutes the most precious human resources contributing to social and economic progress of any nation. Though there is considerable vagueness in the definition of youth and terms like adolescents, youth and young adults which are often used interchangeably. However, World Health Organization (WHO) defines 'adolescence' as the second decade of life from 10 to 19 years, "youth" as those who are in 15-24 years' age group and these two overlapping age groups constitute "young people" covering the age group of 10-24 years (WHO, 2013). As per the National Youth Policy (2014), the age group of 15-29 years considered as youth, and as per the UNESCO report, the age group of 15-24 years are considered as youth.

India is one of the largest demographic countries in this world, with 22.1 percent of youth available in the country. Young people are the nation's future and investment in their development is critical. Youth in the age group of 15-29 years comprise 27.5 percent of the population. At present, about 34 percent of India's Gross National Income (GNI) is contributed by the youth, aged 15-29 years (Paramasivan & Kumaresan, 2016).

Truly, the youth are the most important and dynamic segment of the population in any country. India is witnessing a historic demographic shift and ability to find its rightful place in the community of nations depends upon how well India as a nation, can harness the latent power of the young people of the country. However, there exists a huge potential to increase the contribution of this class of the nation's citizenry by increasing their labour force participation and their productivity (Paramasivan & Kumaresan, 2016).

Adolescents constitute the population in the age group of 10 to 19 years. It is a transitional phase characterized by physical, physiological and psycho-social development ranging from puberty to adulthood. Worldwide, there are more than 1.2 billion adolescents who indicate that roughly one in every six persons is an adolescent (UNICEF, 2012). In India, about 2 percent of total population is adolescent which constitutes about 243 million adolescents (Government of India, 2014). These adolescents are the future of the nation, thus forming a major demographic and economic force.

This period of adolescence further comprises of three phases i.e. early adolescence (11-14 years), middle adolescence (15-17 years) and late adolescence (18-21 years) (Stang & Story, 2005). Young adults are the individuals in the age group of 20 to 24 years (Jekielek & Brown, 2005). The National Youth Policy of India (2003) defines the youth population as those in the age group of 15 to 35 years (Planning Commission Report, 2008).

Adolescence, the most crucial period of life, is a phase of significant physical, physiological, sexual, psychological and behavioural changes with corresponding changes in social interactions and relationships. Adolescents have specific needs which vary with gender, life circumstances and socio-economic conditions. They face many challenges like poverty, lack of access to health care services, unsafe environments etc. It is also a period of preparation for undertaking greater responsibilities like familial, social, cultural and economic issues during adult life.

Thus, adolescence is a period of opportunities that prepares them for a healthy and productive adulthood and to reduce the possibility of health-related issues in the adulthood. Adolescence is a transitional phase accompanied by a myriad of biological changes occurring during puberty which include an increase in height and weight along with changes in body proportions as well as body composition, completion of skeletal growth accompanied by an increase in skeletal mass, menarche followed by sexual maturation. The succession of these events during puberty is generally consistent among the adolescents which are often influenced by gender, age of onset of menarche, its duration along with the other individual variations.

These physical and sexual changes during adolescence are also accompanied by significant stress on young people and those around them while influencing and thus affecting their relationships with the peers and adults. It is also an age of impulsivity accompanied by vulnerability, influenced by peer groups and media that result in changes in perception and practice and characterized by decision making skills/abilities along with acquisition of new emotional, cognitive and social skills (Stang & Story, 2005).

Young People's Health Is Vital and Crucial

Mostly youth is considered to be the healthiest period of life. However, as per WHO estimates, an estimated 2.6 million young people, aged 10 to 24 years, die each year and a much greater number of young people suffer from illnesses which hinder their ability to grow and develop to their full genetic potential. WHO estimates further indicate that roughly two-thirds of premature deaths and one-third of the total morbidity among adults are adverse outcome of conditions or behaviours initiated during adolescence e.g. tobacco use, physical inactivity, high risk sexual behaviours, injury and violence among other such conditions (WHO, 2011).

Although youth is generally considered healthy period of life, various significant public health problems, social behaviours and issues either start or peak during this period (Adolescent Health-Healthy People, 2013). Most of these issues are related to human and social interactions in complex environments that precipitate such behaviours. Developmental transition from childhood to adulthood makes them vulnerable particularly to environmental, contextual or surrounding influences (Mulye, Park, Nelson, Adams, Irwin, & Brindis, 2009).

Review of environmental factors that can promote or adversely affect the young people's health and well-being include family, peer group, school, neighbourhood, community and societal cues (Adolescent Health-Healthy People, 2013). Findings of reported literature reveal the high prevalence of morbidity and mortality among this young population due to varied personal, social, and environmental factors leading to lifestyle changes, encompassing both communicable and non-communicable diseases and injuries suffered by this population.

A significant proportion of this young population is undergoing the conditions that adversely affect their growth and development thus resulting in high incidence of morbidity and mortality rates, which reveal an increasing trend in the coming times. Some of the major health related issues among this young population include under-nutrition and over-nutrition, non-communicable diseases, high risk sexual behaviours, violence, accidents and injuries, common mental and emotional disorders like depression, stress and anxiety, suicidal tendencies and increased suicidal death rates. Most of such conditions can be attributed to ongoing nutritional, epidemiological and environmental conditions affecting the lifestyle pattern of this young population.

The lifestyle pattern during adolescent period determines the current health status of adolescents as well as the risk for developing some chronic diseases in adulthood (Adolescent Health Services, 2013). A significant reduction in the mortality and morbidity of communicable, maternal and neonatal disorders since the year 1990 due to concerted and integrated efforts has led to a shift in focus towards the health, safety and survival of the young people (Gururaj, 2013).

Thus, it is crucial to understand the health problems of this population, processes and mechanisms that affect their health and well-being, to identify the interventions, strategic and approaches that protect their health and development as well as to implement the policies and programmes initiated by the governmental and non-governmental organizations (Collins, 2013).

Global Scenario

The health of young people has been largely neglected in global public health because this age group is wrongfully perceived as healthy. Hence, opportunities for prevention of disease and injury in this age group are not fully exploited.

A review of global scenario of adolescent health reveals that out of more than 1.2 billion adolescents worldwide, about 1.3 million adolescents died from preventable or treatable causes during the year 2012, as per WHO reports (WHO, 2014). About 15 percent of global maternal mortality occurs among adolescent population (Abouzahr, 2013). An increasing trend of adolescent obesity has also been reported due to a transition in the diet and activity pattern (Popkin, 2004).

It has been found that nearly 35 percent of the global burden of diseases has their roots in adolescence. Road traffic accidents and injuries is the leading cause of deaths among adolescents (WHO, 2014). Injuries and neuropsychiatric disorders were the major issues among adolescents. Half of all mental health disorders in adulthood start by 14 years of age, while most such cases are undetected and untreated (WHO, 2014).

In the South East Asian Region (SEAR), unipolar depressive disorders among females and road traffic accidents and injuries among males were the major health concerns which are at the top of the health problems suffered by adolescents. AIDS has emerged as a third leading cause of Disability Adjusted Life Years (DALY's) among adolescents in the last decade (WHO, 2014). These issues need to be addressed for the wellbeing of adolescents.

The total number of incident DALYs in those aged, 10 to 24 years, was about 236 million, representing 15·5% of total DALYs for all age groups. Africa had the highest rate of DALYs for this age group, which was 2·5 times greater than in high-income countries (208 *vs.* 82 DALYs per 1000 population). Across regions, DALY rates were 12% higher in girls than in boys between 15 and 19 years (137 *vs.* 153). Worldwide, the three main causes of YLDs for 10–24-year-olds were neuropsychiatric disorders (45%), unintentional injuries (12%), and infectious and parasitic diseases (10%). The main risk factors for incident DALYs in 10 to 24-year-olds were alcohol (7% of DALYs), unsafe sex (4%), iron deficiency (3%), lack of contraception (2%), and illicit drug use (2%) (Gore, Bloem, George, Ferguson, Véronique, Coffey, Sawyer, & Mathers, 2011).

Although progress has been made since the year 1994 International Conference on Population and Development, adolescents still continue to be disproportionately burdened by threats to their sexual and reproductive health (Bearinger, Sieving, Ferguson, & Sharma, 2007). The ICPD Program of Action further describes services included under the umbrella of sexual and reproductive health services (SRHS), such as family-planning counseling and services; prenatal and postnatal care and delivery; abortion services and post abortion care; treatment and prevention of reproductive tract and sexually transmitted diseases and infections including HIV; and information and counseling about human sexuality.

Problem Status in India

In India, there is general a paucity of health-related data, especially among people in adolescent age group i.e. between 10 to18 years. Until now, National Health Statistics of India has focused mainly on under-five age group especially on the issues of their mortality and morbidity. One of the areas of health related research that has been bypassed concerns the health and nutritional status of adolescents especially girls, who are parents of the future generation.

However, the picture of adolescent health status in India is not different from other parts of the world. India has the largest adolescent population in the world. About 21 percent of total Indian population comprises of adolescents which constitutes about 243 million adolescents (Government of India, 2014).

Physical Health

The physical health status of Indian adolescent population, as revealed by National Family Health Survey (NFHS-3) data, shows that in the age group of 15 to19 years, 47 percent girls and 58 percent boys were thin, 56 percent girls and 30 percent boys were anaemic, 2.4 percent girls and 31.7 percent boys were overweight and 2 out of every 1000 adolescent girls and 1 out of every1000 adolescent boys suffered from diabetes. They were also highly prone for eating disorders like anorexia nervosa or binge eating disorders due to body dissatisfaction and depression (Sivagurunathan, UmaDevi, Rama, & Gopalakrishnan, 2015).

The general health status of the Particularly Vulnerable Tribal Groups (PVTG's) is also not satisfactory as the ICMR report says that,

Analysis of health indices of the tribal population in Odisha are worse than the national average: Infant mortality rate is 84.2; mortality rate under five is 126.6 per thousand children, underweight is 55.9 percent, anaemia in children is 59.8 percent, children with acute respiratory tract infection is 22.4 percent; children with dysentery and diarrhoea is 21.1 percent and women suffering from anaemia is 64.9 per 1000. A high incidence of malnutrition has also been documented in the tribal dominated districts of Odisha. (ICMR, 2003)

The scenario may be almost same for most of the PVTG's and the tribes of Madhya Pradesh and Chhattisgarh are also exhibiting the same picture (Damayanti & Chakma, 2003-2004). The situations of the Baigas population are also very bad: high mortality rate and almost one of the highest infant mortality rate, high level of infectious diseases, under nutrition, delayed menarchae are prevalent among this population (Sahani, 2009).

The disease profile varies across the areas and populations. Among the prevalent diseases; malaria, tuberculosis, respiratory tract infection, diarrhoeal disorders, skin infections including leprosy and iron deficiency anaemias mostly among women and children are the major diseases reported. The exposure of hepatitis infection was also reported from Andaman and Nicobar Islands: 18.5 percent, 48.5 percent and 48 percent for the Great Andamanese, the Onges and the Jarawas respectively, while all the tested Shompens also show the positive result. The virus is endemic in nature, having harmful effect which is very less in comparison to other populations (Murhekar, Chakravarty, Murhekar, Banerjee, & Sehgal, 2006).

The main issue of concern is hereditary haematological disorders, though sizeable data is lacking but the available information is indicating a way towards much alarming situation. The incidence of sickle cell haemoglobin (carrier) is found to even more than 30 percent among the Irular and Paniyan, and more than 22 percent among the Baigas. Similarly, G-6-PD deficiency is observed among the Kutia Khond up to 15 percent of the population. The frequency of thalassaemia gene is found upto 7 per cent among the Lodha. Since, most of the PVTG's practiced endogamy, i.e., marriage within the same community; it may have much more effect on their offsprings (Sahani, 2009).

While adolescents generally enjoy good health compared with other age groups, they face particular health risks, which may be detrimental not only for their immediate future but for the rest of their lives. Estimates and data clearly show that adolescent ill health and death constitute a large portion of the global burden of disease and, therefore, need special attention.

Nutritional Status

There is a methodological debate for assessing malnutrition through haemoglobin and nutritional anthropometry, particularly among the children but Chhotray (2003-04) showed that the particularly vulnerable tribal groups are in critical situation like the Bondo, Didayi, Juang and Kutia Khonds of Odisha in 16 percent, 19 percent, 25.1 percent and 26.6 percent population respectively based on Gomez's classification of malnutrition. The frequency of malnourishment varies and it is 66 percent among the population of 6 to15 years age -group in Mayurbhanj and Sundargarh district while it is 89.4 percent and 88.9 percent among the Langia Sauria and Kutia Khond respectively in Rayagada district.

The adults also correspond to the lower age-groups among the communities like the Khond, Gadaba, Porja, Bondo, Kamar, Kolam, etc., who are showing very serious and critical undernourishment situation. The Kamar community is showing lowest body mass index as well as mid-upper-arm circumference which definitely indicate that they are under the very critical situation. On the other hand, the hunter-gatherer groups of Andaman Islands under the care of Government agency are showing another side of the intervention, especially in nutritional aspect, showing a high prevalence of overweight, though they are short statured people but showing higher value (Sahani 2003; Rao, Sugunan, & Sehgal, 2002).

Recent nutritional studies show that there is reduction of severe malnourished category among the PVTG's in comparison to their past data. The majority of the Bondo, Didayi, Khond and Juang of Odisha had different grades of anaemia as an important clinical manifestation, as per the WHO classification. The severe anaemia (Hb<7g/dl) ranged from 0.6 to 2.3 percent, moderate (Hb 7-9g/dl) from 7.4 to 13.6 percent and mild (Hb 9-11g/dl) from 30.7 to 48.2 percent of the population. Anaemia was more common among females than males. The study also reveals that 85 percent of the Paudi Bhuyan, 40 percent of the Abhuj Maria, 29 percent of the Birhor and 42.2 percent of the Baigas have severe anaemia. An appropriate intervention resulted in the reduction of worm infestation and improvement of anaemia status is 51.2 percent and 34.8 percent of individuals respectively (Chhotray, 2003-04).

The high infant mortality rate, less life expectancy, high prevalence of anaemia due to worm infestation are indicating that the health status are not so good among the PVTG's. For instance, Ali (1980) reported that the bronchitis, asthma, influenza, cough and cold, malaria is very common among the Kutia Khonds of Orissa. There are 21.36 percent sickle cell Haemoglobin and 16 cases of G-6-PD (from 103 tested cases) among them. But sickling has not been reported by Ali among the Dongaria Khond. Acute shortage of food and malnutrition along with associated diseases, Vitamin A and B and iron deficiency among the Chenchus of Andhra Pradesh have been reported. Their maternity ratio is 3.67, mean number of living children per women is 2.66 and survival ratio is 0.72 for all age groups. For 40 years and above age groups, their maternity ratio is 5.70, mean number of living children per women is 3.81 and survival ratio is 0.67. Their mortality rate below one year is 11.66 and below 15 years is 26.13 per 1000 livebirths.

Mukherjee and Nandy (1986) reported malaria, dysentery, stomachache, headache, eye problems, bronchitis, skin diseases among the Asurs. Another study reported body built index among the Padhar of which 30.39 percent is bad, 25.49 percent is very weak and 24.51 percent is weak. According to pelidisi index, 16.67 percent has distinctly low status of nutrition, 20.59 percent has mild under nutrition and 42.16 percent is normal among them.

The Khonds of Odisha almost retain the traditional way of life and are still in the stage of subsistence economy. The different types of foods consumed by the Khondhs are much less than the ICMR standards. The average intake of calories of an adult Khondh is 2084 kcal. which is also less than the ICMR standards. The average adult consumption unit is 4.7 per family. Both weight–for-height and weight-for-age measurements show that the Khondhs are underweight and are in the state of undernutrition. The weight-for-height show 4.76 percent males and 9.30 percent female are beyond 20 percent weight-for-height, while 9.33 percent female and 37.02 percent male have weight-for-height between 10-20 percent. The weight-for-age status depicts that 2.38 percent males are beyond 20 percent of the reference and 5.95 percent between 10-15 percent, while females are showing 10.47 percent frequencies beyond 20 percent and 38.47 percent are between 10 to 20 percent for weight-for-age status (Bulliyya, Mohapatra, Kerketta, Das, & Jangid, 2000-2001).

Pande and Kumar (2004-2005) tried to assess the prevalence of goitre in Baiga tribe taking into consideration the prevalence of iodine deficiency disorder. School children from Baigachak area were also examined for goiter and iodine deficiency. Clinically, iodine deficiency was seen in 83 individuals out of 447 individuals. Majority of the patients were in the age group of 15-44 years followed by 5-14 years' age group. Iodine deficiency seemed to be more prevalent in females.

Damayanti and Chakma (2003-04) studied an ongoing project and 40 percent of the sample has been covered for anthropometry, socio-economic parameters and dietary intake. The anthropometric data reveals that there are no significant differences between tribal adolescents and non-tribal adolescents with respect to height and weight. But with respect to height, girls are taller than boys up to the age of 13-14 years and then boys overtook the girls and finally, boys are 11cm to 15cm taller than girls at 17-18 years. With respect to weight also, tribal adolescent girls are heavier than boys up to the age of 16 years and then boys overtook the girls in the 17-18 years' age group and finally boys are 5-10 kg heavier than girls. The anaemia is the major problem followed by goiter. This observation is based on the clinical signs. There is no difference in the prevalence of nutritional deficiency signs between tribal and non-tribals.

It is also reported that the *Kutia Khond* women are 3-4 cm. shorter in height whereas the body weight deficit is 13.8-14.4 kg (35.3-39 kgm) than the respective age group of males in Phulbani district (Patel, 1985). The range of BMI varies between males (20.8-21.8 Kg/mt2) and females (15.8-19.8 Kg/mt2). Corresponding to ICMR height standards, the proportion of women with weight deficiency is greater i.e. 72 percent as compared to men (32%).

Similar observations were made in Andhra Pradesh where the *Khond* women (20-40 years) are deficient for both height (3.8%) and weight (24.01%) with a BMI of 17.7 Kg/mt2 (Kupputhai & Mallika, 1993). It is also observed that mean height and weight of the elderly *Khond* women are 144 cm and 37 kgm. Iron deficiency anaemia accounted for 94 percent of the elderly *Khond* women (Bulliyya, Mohapatra, Kerketta, Das, & Jangid, 2000-2001).

Another interesting study was conducted on the nutritional status of the *Kamars* of Madhya Pradesh (Gangopadhyay, 2006) which revealed that the consumption of all the nutrients, except vitamin B1 is lower than the ICMR recommendations. It was mentioned that only 25 percent of households consume more than 2501 kilocalorie per day (ICMR recommendation is 2875 Kilo calorie/day). The *Kamar* families in general consume lesser amount of calories than actually required. The mean BMI of both the sexes revealed, "mildly undernourished" nutritional status among the studied *Kamar* population.

A survey of 227 families of the *Santals* and 494 families of the *Paharias* was carried out to evaluate the consequences of genetic load in terms of foetal and infant deaths. Significantly higher percentage of foetal loss was observed among the *Pahariyas* (22.5%) in comparison to the *Santals* (16.5%). This loss was recorded highest during 5-19 weeks of pregnancies in both the tribes. Maximum foetal loss occurred during 0 to 7 days and 8 to 27 days. Among the demographic factors, only age of the mothers had profound effect in foetal and infant deaths. During post-natal period, the infant deaths may be due to various problems including weaning of the baby with inadequate and improper supplementation of food. The baby is exposed freely to the outside world. The sudden exposure subjects the babies to the risk of contact with unhealthy persons and environment (Choudhary & Adhikari, 1997).

Psycho-Social Health

Besides these physical and nutritional health problems, mental health problems are one of the most important but neglected issues among adolescent population in India. Mortality and morbidity due to mental disorders in adolescents have increased and topped in the recent years. In India, suicide rate among adolescents is higher than in any other age groups. Findings of a study reported that 40 percent of suicide deaths in men and 56 percent of suicide deaths in women occurred in 15 to 29 years of age (Patel, Ramasundarahettige, Vijayakumar, Thakur, Gajalakshmi, & Gururaj, 2012).

A study from Goa conducted on 16 to 24 years old adolescents revealed that 3.9 percent of youth reported suicidal behaviours, with females being four times more prone to suicidal behaviours than their male counterparts. This suicidal behaviour was independently associated with factors like absenteeism, independent decision making, premarital sex, sexual abuse, physical abuse from parents and mental disorders (Pillai, Andrews, & Patel, 2009).

The prevalence rate of child and adolescent psychiatric disorders in the community has been found to be 6.46 percent and in schools, it was found to be 23.33 percent. However, the reporting systems of psychiatric disorders in children are found to be inadequate (Malhotra & Patra, 2014; Rani & Karunanidhi, 2010). From the above studies, it is evident that a considerable proportion of adolescents have psycho-social problems.

During the years 2001-03, nearly 20 percent of the total deaths in the 5 to 29 years age groups were reported to be due to unintentional injuries in India (Jagnoor Suraweera, Keay, Ivers, Thakur, & Jha, 2012). About 77.5 percent of road-traffic accidents and deaths were reported in Delhi among adolescents due to their risky behaviours (Sharma, Grover, & Chaturvedi, 2007).

Substance abuse is yet another serious problem among adolescents in India as they are ignorant about its adverse effects. National Family Health Survey (NFHS–3) data shows that in the age group 15 to 19 years, about 11 percent of adolescent boys and one percent of adolescent girls had consumed alcohol, out of which, 3 percent consumed it daily. Findings of the survey revealed that about 29 percent boys and 4 percent girls used some kind of tobacco. The average age at initiation of tobacco use was as early as 12.3 years and alcohol usage was 13.6 years among adolescents (Tikoo, Dhawan, Pattanayak, & Chopra, 2013). It was also revealed that about 11 percent of cannabis users were introduced to it before the age of 15 years (Ministry of Health and Family Welfare, Government of India, 2014). Initiating cannabis at this age is strongly associated with the development of Schizophrenia spectrum disorders in adulthood (Anglin, Corcoran, Brown, Chen, Lighty, & Brook, 2012).

Childhood and adolescence are crucial periods for laying the foundations for healthy development and good mental health. Poor mental health in childhood is associated with health and social problems such as school failure, delinquency and substance abuse and increases the risk of poverty and other adverse outcomes in adulthood.

Sexual and Reproductive Health

Besides, adolescents suffer from varied problems related to their sexual and reproductive health. As per NFHS–3 data, 2.7 percent boys and 8 percent girls reported sexual debut before the age of 15 years and most of the sexual activity happens in the context of marriage, thus leading to early pregnancy and its adverse outcomes. Even though contraceptive awareness is 94 percent among girls aged 15 to19 years, only 23 percent of the married and 18 percent of the sexually active unmarried girls in this group used a contraceptive once at least (National Family Health Survey (NFHS-3), 2005–06). All the three NFHS findings show almost an equal prevalence (59.1 percent, 59.8 percent and 58.2 percent) of pregnant and mothered adolescents and there is a steady increase in percentage of first pregnancy among adolescents (11.7 percent, 12.4 percent and 14.4 percent) over the recent years due to early marriage and low contraceptive usage by pregnant adolescents.

Sexual abuse is yet another issue of concern for both adolescent girls and boys. These problems mostly go unnoticed as the victim suffers in silence because of fear and social stigma. This indirectly affects the physical health, mental health and the academic performance (Patel & Andrew, 2001).

In India, adolescent fertility rate contributes to 17 percent to the total fertility rate and about 14 percent of births in women, aged below 20 years, are unplanned (Ministry of Health and Family Welfare, Government of India, 2014). Early and unplanned adolescent pregnancies are the contributing risk factors for adverse pregnancy outcomes like maternal mortality, low birth weight babies, early neonatal deaths, eclampsia and congenital malformation (Ganchimeg, 2014).

In addition, 34 percent of ever-married adolescent girls in the age group of 15 to 19 years reported that they suffered physical, emotional or sexual violence inflicted by their partner (Ministry of Health and Family Welfare, Government of India, 2014). There is a remarkable decline in these rates as the age of marriage rises. Moreover, early marriage also carries the risk of subjecting girls to all forms of violence.

In India, it has been found that only 19 percent adolescent girls and 35 percent adolescent boys had comprehensive knowledge about HIV/AIDS. Only 15 percent young men and women in the age group of 15 to 24 years reported that they received family life or sex education (Ministry of Health and Family Welfare, Government of India, 2014).

Eventually due to inadequate knowledge, they are at a greater risk of exposure to unprotected sex, unethical sexual practice and STI's. In the age group of 15 to19 years, among those who had sexual intercourse, 10.5 percent of girls and 10.8 percent of boys reported having STI's or symptoms of STI's and 0.07 percent of girls and 0.01 percent of boys were found to be HIV positive (National Family Health Survey (NFHS-3), 2005–06). The probable reason could be lack of awareness regarding transmission of STI's among adolescents in India. Due to this, such diseases are often undisclosed, left untreated leading to complications like infertility, pelvic inflammatory disease and cancer, besides it being considered a social stigma.

With such a scenario, there is a strong need for public health community to identify, prepare, integrate and implement activities that help to promote health and healthy lifestyles of young people and establish mechanisms for delivery of population-based interventions along with measuring its impact. There is also a need to conduct baseline surveys and good quality researches so that suitable intervention programmes can be designed to cater to the needs of this vulnerable population. Strategic investments in nutrition, sexual and reproductive health, education and employment are critical for healthy growth and all around development of adolescents and these programmes need to be monitored and evaluated periodically for their efficacy and effectiveness using public health approaches.

Among various dimensions of adolescent health care, the first and foremost priority should be in the health and nutrition sectors with proper planning. The planners must have adequate knowledge regarding the needs of the community and should have a lot of research exposure of the traditional society. Since the nutritional intervention of the globe shows that while reducing under-nutrition by intervention, exact proportion of the over-nutrition emerges out, which has more disastrous effect than the under nutrition (WHO, 1995).

Adolescent Health Care System in India

India is the world largest population particularly youth population, as per 2011 census report. Youth can make or mar any society. Youth can promote social and economic development as well as sustainable growth in India. Youth in Indian situation offers a roadmap for programmes and priorities that aim to address the issues and challenges in order to fully meet the needs of youth in a rapidly globalizing world as well as enable the country to reap the benefits of the demographic dividend.

In India, all the existing Maternal and Child Health (MCH) programmes are an important means of reducing nutritional deficiencies during pregnancy through food and iron supplementation. These programmes, however, do not provide enough supplementation to overcome pre-existing deficits in women's nutritional status.

Attention to improve the nutritional status of adolescent girls, before the reproductive years begin, can ensure adequate pre-pregnancy weight and adequate physical development, which can reduce maternal mortality due to obstructed labour and reduce infant mortality. In addition, a focus on adolescent nutrition will help girls to realize their educational opportunities in a better way and prepare them for future work demands. There is perhaps no other segment of society less served at the moment and some more deserving, in which a substantial investment will give greater yield.

Though Adolescent Friendly Health Services (AFHS) based adolescent clinics are said to address all the health needs of adolescents, the delivery of services mainly targets reproductive and sexual health and all other issues are not adequately focused. Even with this great focus on ARSH, NFHS data shows no significant decrease in adolescent pregnancy. In fact, there is an increasing trend in first pregnancy in adolescent and the birthrate in the age group 15 to 19 y is still 31.5 per thousand adolescent girls, which is high for the efforts and inputs given by the health system (SRS Statistical Report, 2012).

Adolescent health services are not comprehensive, so many schemes exist but these schemes are placed under different ministries and some of the schemes provide the same services as others which may result in unnecessary duplication. In the year 2014, Ministry of Health & Family Welfare (MoHFW), launched a comprehensive programme (Rashtriya Kishor Swasthya Karyakram), but similar services provided by MoHFW and other ministries are not going to be terminated.

To avoid such confusions and to be cost effective, all the services for adolescents should come under a single program. It is also essential to develop a screening tool specific for Indian adolescents. This has been already implemented in United States by National Adolescent and Young Adult Health Information Centre, University of California (UCSF Division of Adolescent and Young Adult Medicine, 2014). Innovating such tools based on our requirements can be very useful in diagnosing diseases and to search for and eliminate any risk factors as early as possible.

Thus, there is a need to call for the development of programmes in this country, especially for young adolescent girls that will assure that they grow into healthy women, knowledgeable about themselves and their future goals and responsibilities, aware of the world around them, its opportunities and challenges and be able to be self-respecting and independent adults within the society. The benefits of all these efforts will undoubtedly enhance not only their own lives but be an appropriate legacy to the next generation and even those beyond.

All the adolescent health programmes being implemented by various ministries under the initiative of Government of India target diverse adolescent health problems. However, these programmes are fragmentary at present and there is no comprehensive and integrated programme addressing all developmental needs and concerns of adolescents. Moreover, the access and availability of health care services are severely limited.

However, to achieve this objective of wholesome adolescent health, there is an urgent need to have a multi-dimensional approach covering all the adolescent health problems with special emphasis on physical and mental health, sexual and reproductive health, behaviour change, communication towards healthy lifestyle and positive social environment to acquire life skills.

This multi-dimensional approach must focus on the strategy that there should be adolescent friendly clinics need to address the issues and concerns pertaining to adolescent health and wellbeing. These clinics should focus to achieve universal coverage of the target population. Health of adolescents should be monitored on regular basis which could be an effective tool for detection and treatment of existing diseases and to prevent the occurrence of any new disease. Empowering the adolescents through life skill education and involving them in decisions that affect them and facilitate them with every opportunity for developing into a successful adult. Offering such opportunities to the growing adolescents gives them a chance to build a safe, happy, healthy and productive nation in the future.

REFERENCES

Abouzahr, C. (2013). *Women's health meeting: trends and projections for mortality and morbidity*. Available from: http://icpdbeyond2014.org/uploads/browser/files/maternal_mortality_trends_and_projections.pdf

Adolescent health and development. (n.d.). WHO Regional 1. Office for South-East Asia. Available from: http://www.searo.who.int/entity/child_adolescent/topics/adolescent_health/en/index.html

Adolescent Health-Healthy People. (2013). Available from: http://www.healthypeople.gov/2020/topicsobjectives2020/overview.aspx?topicid=2#Ref_03

Adolescent Health Services. (2013). *Missing Opportunities*. Available from: http://books.nap.edu/openbook.php?record_id=12063&page=1

Ali, A. (1980). Health and genetic problems of Kutia Kondhs of Bulubaru village, Phulbani district, Orissa. The Newsletter, 1(2), 103-114.

Anglin, D. M., Corcoran, C. M., Brown, A. S., Chen, H., Lighty, Q., Brook, J. S., & Cohen, P. R. (2012). Early cannabis use and schizotypal personality disorder symptoms from adolescence to middle adulthood. *Schizophrenia Research, 137*(1-3), 45–49. doi:10.1016/j.schres.2012.01.019 PMID:22325079

Bearinger, L. H., Sieving, R. E., Ferguson, J., & Sharma, V. (2007). Global perspectives on the sexual and reproductive health of adolescents: Patterns, prevention and potential. *Lancet, 369*(9568), 1220–1231. doi:10.1016/S0140-6736(07)60367-5 PMID:17416266

Bulliyya, G., Mohapatra, S. S. S., Kerketta, A. S., Das, R. K., & Jangid P. K. (2001). *Assessment of health and nutritional profile among the elderly population of Orissa Primitive tribes.* Annual Report. Regional Medical Research Centre, Bhubaneswar.

Chhotray, G. P. (2004). *Studies on Nutrition.* Annual Report 2003-04, Regional Medical Research Centre, Bhubaneshwar.

Choudhary, R. P., & Adhikari, D. (1997). Foetal and infant mortality in two tribes of Rajmahal hills of Bihar. *Journal of Human Ecology (Delhi, India), 8*(1), 43–49. doi:10.1080/09709274.1997.11907234

Collins, P. Y., Insel, T. R., Chockalingam, A., Daar, A., & Maddox, Y. T. (2013). Grand challenges in global mental health: Integration in research, policy, and practice. *PLoS Medicine, 1*(4), e1001434. doi:10.1371/journal.pmed.1001434 PMID:23637578

Damayanti, K., & Chakma, T. (2004). *Nutritional status of adolescents in tribal areas of Madhya Pradesh. Chapter 2: Nutrition.* Annual Report. Regional Medical Research Centre for Tribals (ICMR), Jabalpur.

Ganchimeg, T., Ota, E., Morisaki, N., Laopaiboon, M., Lumbiganon, P., Zhang, J., ... Mori, R. (2014). Pregnancy and childbirth outcomes among adolescent mothers: A World Health Organization multi-country study. *BJOG, 121*(s1), 40–48. doi:10.1111/1471-0528.12630 PMID:24641534

Gangopadhyay, S. (2006). Nutritional Status of the Kamar of Madhya Pradesh. In P. Dash Sharma (Ed.), *Anthropology of Primitive Tribes in India* (pp. 412–430). New Delhi: Sterling Publication.

Gore, F. M., Bloem, P. J. N., George, C. P., Ferguson, J., Véronique, J., Coffey, C., ... Mathers, C. D. (2011). Global burden of disease in young people aged 10–24 years: A systematic analysis. *Lancet, 377*(9783), 2093–2102. doi:10.1016/S0140-6736(11)60512-6 PMID:21652063

Government of India. (2014). Ministry of Health and Family Welfare. Available from: https://www.dropbox.com/s/0oj4p422y7st4ku/RKSK%20Strategy%20Handbook.pdf

Gururaj, G. (2013). Injury prevention and care: an important public health agenda for health, survival and safety of children. *Indian Journal of Pediatrics, 2*(80), S100-8.

ICMR. (2003). Health status of primitive tribes of Orissa. Indian Council of Medical Research Bulletin, 33(10).

Jagnoor, J., Suraweera, W., Keay, L., Ivers, R., Thakur, J., & Jha, P. (2012). Unintentional injury mortality in India, 2005: Nationally representative mortality survey of 1.1 million homes. *BMC Public Health, 12*(1), 487. doi:10.1186/1471-2458-12-487 PMID:22741813

Jekielek, S., & Brown, B. (2005). *The Transition to Adulthood: 4. Characteristics of Young Adults Ages 18 to 24 in America.* Kids count/PRb/Child Trends Report on Census 2000. The Annie Casey Foundation, Population reference bureau, and Child trends, Washington, DC. Available from: http://www.prb.org/pdf05/transitiontoadulthood.pdf

Kupputhai, U., & Mallika, N. (1993). Nutrional status of adult women belonging to Khond, Gadaba and Porja tribes of Andhra Pradesh. *The Indian Journal of Nutrition and Dietetics, 30*(7), 173–179.

Malhotra, S., & Patra, B. (2014). Prevalence of child and adolescent psychiatric disorders in India: A systematic review and meta-analysis. *Child and Adolescent Psychiatry and Mental Health, 8*(1), 22. doi:10.1186/1753-2000-8-22 PMID:25071865

Mukherjee, D. P., & Nandy, S. K. (1986). Anthropology of tribal health- the Cause of the Asur in Neterhat Plateau. In B. Chaudhury (Ed.), *Tribal health: Socio-cultural dimensions* (pp. 247–258). New Delhi: Inter India Publication.

Mulye, T. P., Park, M. J., Nelson, C. D., Adams, S. H., Irwin, C. E. Jr, & Brindis, C. D. (2009). Trends in adolescent and young adult health in the United States. *The Journal of Adolescent Health, 45*(1), 8–24. doi:10.1016/j.jadohealth.2009.03.013 PMID:19541245

Murhekar, M. V., Chakravarty, R., Murhekar, K. M., Banerjee, A., & Sehgal, S. C. (2006). Hepatitis B virus genotypes among the Jarawas: A primitive Negrito tribe of Andaman and Nicobar Islands, India. *Archives of Virology, 151*(8), 1499–1510. doi:10.100700705-006-0737-8 PMID:16514497

National Family Health Survey (NFHS-3). (2006). *India: Volume I.* International Institute for Population Sciences (IIPS) and Macro International. Mumbai: IIPS. Available from: http://www.rchiips.org/nfhs/NFHS-3%20 Data/VOL- 1/India_volume_I_corrected_17oct08.pdf

Pande, P. L., & Kumar, S. (2005). *Assessment of iodine deficiency disorders in Baiga Chak area of district Dindori.* 26 RMRCT Annual Report.

Paramasivan, C., & Kumaresan, K. (2016). Demographic Profile of Youth in India. *SELP Journal of Social Science*, *7*(29), 7–11.

Patel, S. (1985). *Ecology, ethnology and nutrition: A study of Khondh tribals and Tibetan refugees*. Delhi: Mittal Publication.

Patel, V., Ramasundarahettige, C., Vijayakumar, L., Thakur, J., Gajalakshmi, V., Gururaj, G., ... Jha, P. (2012). Suicide mortality in India: A nationally representative survey. *Lancet*, *379*(9834), 2343–2351. doi:10.1016/S0140-6736(12)60606-0 PMID:22726517

Pillai, A., Andrews, T., & Patel, V. (2009). Violence, psychological distress and the risk of suicidal behaviour in young people in India. *International Journal of Epidemiology*, *38*(2), 459–469. doi:10.1093/ije/dyn166 PMID:18725364

Planning Commission. (n.d.). *Report of the Steering committee on Youth Affairs and Sports for the Eleventh Five Year Plan (2007-12)*. Available from: http://planningcommission.nic.in/aboutus/committee/strgrp11/str_yas.pdf

Popkin, B., & Gordon-Larsen, P. (2004). The nutrition transition: worldwide obesity dynamics and their determinants. *International Journal of Obesity*, *28*, 2-9. Available from: http://www.cpc.unc.edu/projects/nutrans/publications/Popkin%20Nutr%20Trans%20IJO%202004.pdf

Population and Development. (1995). *Programme of Action adopted at the International Conference on Population and Development, Cairo*. New York: United Nations, Dept. for Economic and Social Information and Policy Analysis.

Rani, M., & Karunanidhi, S. (2010). Prevalence of depressive symptoms among urban adolescents in South India. *Journal of Indian Association for Child Adolescent Mental Health*, *6*(2), 33–43.

Rao, V. G., Sugunan, A. P., & Sehgal, S. C. (2002). Nutritional status of some tribes of Andaman and Nicobar Islands. *Tribal Health Bulletin*, *8*, 24–33.

Sahani, R. (2003). Nutritional and health status of the Jarawas: A preliminary report. *Journal of the Anthropological Survey of India*, *52*, 47–65.

Sahani, S., & Nandy, S. K. (2013). Particularly Vulnerable Tribal Groups in India: An Overview. *Journal of the Anthropological Survey of India*, *62*(2), 851–865.

Sharma, R., Grover, V., & Chaturvedi, S. (2007). Health-risk behaviours related to road safety among adolescent students. *Indian Journal of Medical Sciences*, *61*(12), 656–662. doi:10.4103/0019-5359.37786 PMID:18174635

Sivagurunathan, C., UmaDevi, R., Rama, R., & Gopalakrishnan, S. (2015). Adolescent Health: Present Status and Its Related Programmes in India. Are We in the Right Direction? *Journal of Clinical and Diagnostic Research*, *9*(3), 1-6.

Stang, J., & Story, M. (2005). Adolescent growth and development. In *Guidelines for adolescent nutrition services*. Minneapolis, MN: Center for Leadership, Education and Training in Maternal and Child Nutrition, Division of Epidemiology and Community Health, School of Public Health, University of Minnesota; Available from: http://www.epi.umn.edu/let/pubs/img/adol_ch1.pdf

Statistical Report, S. R. S. (2012). *SRS Statistical Report Tables, Vital Statistics, Sl. No.12, Ministry of Home Affairs*. Available from: http:// www.censusindia.gov.in/vital_statistics/SRS_Report_2012/12_SRS_statistical_report_ tables_2012.pdf

Tikoo, V., Dhawan, A., Pattanayak, R., & Chopra, A. (2013). *Assessment of Pattern and Profile of Substance Use among Children in India*. Available from: http://www.ncpcr.gov.in/view_file.php?fid=17

UCSF Division of Adolescent and Young Adult Medicine. (2014). *Summary of Recommended Guidelines for Clinical Preventive Services for Young Adults ages 18-26: Risk Factors and Recommended Screening Tests*. Available from: http://nahic.ucsf.edu/wp-content/uploads/2014/04/ FINAL-Screening-Guidelines-4.11.pdf

UNICEF. (2012). *Progress for Children: A report card on adolescents. Socio-demographic profile of adolescents: Number 10 April 2012 UNICEF. Figure: 2.1 Page 6*. Available from: http://www.unicef.org/publications/files/Progress_for_Children_-_No._10_EN_04232012.pdf

World Health Organization. (1995). *Physical Status: the use and interpretation of anthropometry*. WHO Technical Report Series 854. Retrieved from www.andaman.org

World Health Organization. (2014). *Health for world's adolescents: Disability Adjusted Life Years: Combining Mortality and Morbidity*. Available from: http://public.tableausoftware.com/profile/digitalteam#!/vizhome/shared/FPXZ7PPMR

Young people: health risks and solutions. Fact sheet no. 345. 8. (2011). World Health Organization. Available from: http://www.who.int/mediacentre/factsheets/fs345/en/index.html

Chapter 2
Physical Health

ABSTRACT

Though adolescence is relatively a healthier period of life as compared to childhood, several risk factors of adult diseases having their onset during adolescence can be prevented with proper interventions during this period, though with many challenges. Data on the health and nutritional status of adolescents is of vital importance not merely in the context of improving the quality of their lives but also for providing valuable insight into issues that are likely to have profound bearing on the future generations. However, the exclusive data pertaining to the adolescent health issues in Indian scenario is not available as compared to other nations. Hence, the data pertaining to South East Asia region for comparison has been referred to, in which India is a major constituent country. The data about important adolescent health issues in different areas is scarce. Hence, detailed investigation of the incidence and interventions on adolescent health issues is the need of the hour.

KEY FACTS

- Nearly 10 to 30 percent of young people suffer from health impacting behaviours and conditions that need urgent attention of policy makers and public health professionals (Singh & Gururaj, 2014).
- Iron Deficiency Anaemia is the leading cause of Years Lost to Death and Disability among female adolescents during the year 2015 (Sivagurunathan, UmaDevi, Rama, & Gopalakrishnan, 2015).

DOI: 10.4018/978-1-5225-7384-5.ch002

- Obesity has become a colossal epidemic causing serious public health concern and contributes to 2.6 million deaths worldwide every year (WHO, 2005).
- Other major causes of adolescent deaths include diarrhoea and lower respiratory tract infections (LRTI's) which are estimated to be among the top five causes of deaths for 10 to 19-year-old adolescents.

INTRODUCTION

In the growth process of human beings, adolescence occupies a significant period with rapid changes in growth and progressive attainment of adult status. Adolescence is characterized by the onset of major maturational events, principally the spurt in somatic growth and the accompanying appearance of secondary sexual characteristics and the onset of menarche and spermarche in adolescent girls and boys respectively. The growth and maturation timings may be affected by environmental and health factors, though the genetic factors are primarily responsible for the timing of maturation events (Tanner, 1962). Thus, the normal variability in growth at adolescence may be due to genetic and hormonal changes which are environmentally induced (Tanner, 1962; Malina & Bouchard, 1991).

Adolescents are a group of apparently healthy individuals. The health status of an adolescent determines the health status in his/her adulthood. Many serious diseases in adulthood have their roots in adolescence. Also, adolescents face premature mortality due to various reasons that are either preventable or treatable and many more suffer from chronic ill-health and disability.

This young population constitutes one of the precious resources of a country. This phase is characterized by rapid growth and development and is a phase of vulnerability which is often influenced by several intrinsic and extrinsic factors that affect their health and safety. Nearly 10 to 30 per cent of young people suffer from health impacting behaviours and conditions that need urgent attention of policy makers and public health professionals (Singh & Gururaj, 2014).

Nutritional disorders, including malnutrition and over-nutrition, tobacco use, harmful alcohol use, other substance use, high risk sexual behaviours, stress, common mental disorders and injuries especially road traffic injuries, suicides, violence of different types specifically affect this population and have long lasting impact on their health and well-being.

At the individual level, puberty is generally beginning earlier although it has reached a plateau in some industrialized countries and is being delayed in the poorest while the mean age of marriage is rising. These many factors in combination are having an impact on young people's behavior and society's treatment of them with important consequences for their own psychological, physical, mental as well as social health and wellbeing, their future health and longevity and also that of the children born to them. Moreover, they are at a time of life with great energy, creativity and enthusiasm and that if given the right degree of support and opportunity, they are a great resource for the present and future of all societies (Friedman, 1994).

Physical Health Needs

The health needs of the adolescents can be broadly categorized into three major categories- physical, psychological and social. The main physical health issues faced by adolescents include many physical health problems, early pregnancy and childbirth, Human Immune Deficiency Virus/Sexually Transmitted Infection (HIV/STI) and other infectious diseases, violence, unintentional injuries, malnutrition and substance abuse.

Generally, health and nutritional status of adolescent girls is affected by the continuing life cycle; their own conception and growth as a fetus, birth, infancy, childhood, early adolescence, womanhood, marriage and once again conception. The maintenance of such a continuous life cycle is determined largely by the nutritional status of adolescent girls when they are in the 10-18 years' age bracket. Girls in this particular age group have made the transition from the nutritionally vulnerable years of late infancy and late childhood to the threshold of bearing children of their own. In developing countries such as India, where 50 to 65 percent of children below five years of age suffer from various degrees of under-nutrition, the health and nutritional status of adolescent girls have a great bearing on overall child health status, morbidity and mortality rates (Regmi & Adhikari, 1994).

Malnutrition, especially among children and adolescents, is the problem to be solved because adolescence is the precarious juncture between an impoverished childhood and a demanding future. In most of the developing countries including India, adolescent girls face more limited access to nutrition, education and training and are at a higher risk of under-nutrition because of heavy workloads and the demands of pregnancy. The reproductive cycle of pregnancy, childbirth and lactation are nutritionally demanding and adolescent mothers face these demands while they themselves are still growing and developing (Tanner, 1990). The result is often compromised stature or incomplete pelvic growth with consequent risk of maternal death from obstructed labour.

The causes of malnutrition are varied and are country as well as society specific. In developing countries like India, where majority of the population lies below poverty line, access to food may be inadequate due to poverty, seasonal food supplies or inequitable intra-household allocation patterns. In some settings, gender discrimination in the distribution of food within the household may compound the problem. The problem of malnutrition aggravates further due to environmental insanitation causing infectious and parasitic diseases, resulting in acute blood and iron loss, which leads to Iron Deficiency Anaemia (IDA). High rates of iron deficiencies are common among adolescent girls in developing countries (ACC/SCN, 1991). Additionally, iodine deficiency still exists in many areas where National Iodine Prophylaxis Programme has not yet been expanded. Thus, increasing the quality and quantity of food intake is one of the most commonly adopted strategies for improving the nutritional status of this group of population.

Physical Growth Pattern

During adolescence, the nutritional requirements in relation to body size are more. Majority of the adolescent girls do not achieve their full height and weight potential on account of their dietary insufficiencies. The nutritional status, which is often poor during early life, gets worsened as the adolescent growth spurt occurs (Senapati, 1990). Malnutrition during childhood also retards growth and delays the appearance of growth spurt.

A study by Datta Banik (1982) on semi-longitudinal evaluation of Indian children (0 to14 years) among different socio-economic groups revealed that mean height and weight of children of both sexes belonging to higher socio-economic status compared well with 50th percentile height and weight of American children. The 50th percentile height of Indian children from lower socio-economic status corresponded with 25th percentile height of American children. The 50th percentile weight of lower socio-economic status Indian children corresponded with 10th percentile weight of American children. This data reveals that children with good nutrition and belonging to higher socio-economic status are as tall and heavy as American children of the corresponding age, thus indicating that well fed children of different countries grow in a similar pattern in spite of racial differences. Thus, nutritional factor plays a greater role than racial (genetic) factors in influencing growth of children as well as adolescents.

The growth pattern of affluent Indian girls, as reported by Vijayaraghavan and Nutrition Foundation of India (NFI), was found to be practically identical to National Centre for Health Statistics curve up to 12.0 years and deviate considerably after 12 years of age. The findings demonstrated that growth pattern of Indian affluent girls, without any apparent dietary and environmental constraints, was comparable to that of the American girls in the pre-adolescence phase. At the time of growth spurt, i.e. 12 to18 years, the growth of Indian girls slowed down and resulted in a difference of 5 cm in height at the end of 18 years. The entire difference in height, therefore, sets in between 12 to 18 years i.e. the period of adolescence (NFI, 1989).

The reported findings on growth pattern of adolescent girls from rural population of India by National Nutrition Monitoring Beaureu (NNMB) when compared to the data of Indian affluent girls demonstrated an absolute difference of 7 cm in the mean height of adolescent girls and the corresponding difference of 6.5 kg in the mean weight of adolescent girls (NFI, 1989). These findings clearly reflect the adverse effects of environmental constraints on growth of rural adolescent girls in India.

The diminished growth pattern of adolescent girls due to adverse effects of environmental constraints reflects upon interplay of varied reasons, the inadequate and imbalanced diet being one of important reasons. Since adolescence is an intense anabolic period, the requirement for all the nutrients is increased during this period. Forbes (1980) illustrated the biological rationale for recommended increases in intake of several nutrients during adolescence and how these increases in intake of nutrients varied with physiological age by calculating average daily increments in body content of these nutrients over the second decade of life and daily increments at the peak of the growth spurt. It was noted that the daily increments at the peak of the growth spurt were almost double the daily average values for the decade. It was also found that the increments were more highly associated with the physiological age than the chronological age.

While working in a hospital setting in Italy, Agostoni et al. (1994) recommended a balanced intake of the macronutrients (protein, fat and carbohydrates) to prevent the chronic degenerative disorders of adulthood.

The temporal pattern of calorie intake also deserves much attention since it may affect the homeostatic regulation.

Adolescents grow at a greatest rate than any other age group after infancy and accumulate 37 percent of the total bone mass during their growth spurt. Since maximum bone mass is acquired during adolescence, the calcium deposited during adolescence determines the risk of osteoporosis and fractures in adulthood. Bone mass accumulation is dependent on calcium intake, growth and pubertal development, exercise as well as genetic and racial factors. Unfortunately, during this time of tremendous calcium need, most adolescents eat a diet that is very deficient in calcium, thereby adversely affecting their skeletal development.

Other factors contributing to poor bone mineralization include adolescent pregnancy, anorexia nervosa, excessive exercise and various chronic medical conditions. To avoid osteoporosis in later life, adequate dietary calcium intake should be recommended and calcium supplementation considered for all adolescents.

In addition, to meet the increased iron needs of the expanding red cell mass and myoglobin in the newly gained muscle tissues, adolescent girls have a further increased iron requirement up to 15 percent to compensate for the menstrual blood losses (National Research Council, 1989).

Adolescents often show disorders of dietary behavior, thereby predisposing them to both obesity and anorexia. Dietary interventions in this age group should promote the regular consumption of breakfast, a balanced intake of animal and vegetable foods and an increased calcium supply to maximize bone density. Dairy products, vegetables and enriched cereals constitute the basis of a good diet for adolescents to meet their needs for growth and for subsequent good health (National Institute of Nutrition, 1998).

Nutritional Health Status

Nutritional requirements are higher during adolescence than any other period of life because of rapid growth spurt marked by puberty during this period. Inadequate dietary intake at this age leads to stunted growth and delayed sexual maturation (Stang & Story, 2005). Lots of junk food products are promoted by celebrities with catchy advertisements leading to adaptation of unhealthy food habits. Media influences the diet and lifestyle among adolescents and leads to nutritional disorders by making them sedentary and giving false hopes. Habits like dieting and exercising inspired by a media celebrity cannot be taken as a positive impact, often they do it in an incorrect way and consume low quality protein supplements without proper guidance of dieticians or nutritionists which may often lead to complications like renal failure etc. Instead of taking balanced diet, they starve and end up in anorexia nervosa. These issues can be reduced to a great extent by routine screening and assessment of health and nutritional status of adolescents and nutrition education so as to enable them to maintain good health and nutritional status.

The findings of author's research on nutrient adequacy of selected population of rural adolescent girls from Haryana in India revealed that all the macro- as well as micro-nutrients were deficient to the extent of 50 percent in their diets, except for thiamin and phosphorus, which were found to be adequate. Results of the study revealed that calorie deficit was to the extent of 48.4 percent and 44.5 percent of Recommended Dietary Allowances (RDA) among 10 to 12 years and 13 to 15 years' age group respectively which was significantly reduced by 29.4 percent and 25 percent of RDA respectively in younger and older girls as a result of 6 months of dietary supplementation (Nanda, 2001).

The deficit in Protein intake was to the tune of 47.2 percent and 50.5 percent of RDA among 10 to 12 and 13 to15 years old adolescent girls respectively which reduced significantly by 24 percent and 20.2 percent of RDA respectively after dietary supplementation given for 6 months. Likewise, the fat deficit decreased significantly by 27.5 percent and 14 percent of RDA respectively among young and older adolescent girls after dietary supplementation. Carbohydrate deficit also reduced significantly by 27.4 percent and 25.1 of RDA percent in younger and older girls respectively as a result of dietary supplementation (Nanda, 2001).

The adequacy of iron was found to be 71.6 percent of RDA among 10 to12 years old pre-menarcheal girls as compared to 51.1 percent of RDA among 13-15 years old adolescent girls who had just attained menarche. Iron adequacy improved to 113 percent and 84 percent of RDA respectively in pre-menarcheal and menarcheal girls as a result of dietary supplementation which was further improved to 218.5 percent and 155 percent of RDA repectively in pre-menarcheal and menarcheal girls after iron and folic acid supplementation in addition to dietary supplementation (Nanda, 2001).

Adequacy of vitamin C intake also improved 11.8 and 7.4 fold respectively among younger and older adolescents as a result of supplementation, thereby improving the absorption and utilization of iron in their bodies. Dietary supplementation also reduced the calcium deficit significantly by 23.8 percent and 21.6 percent of RDA respectively in younger and older adolescent girls (Nanda, 2001).

Though the deficit of water soluble vitamin B2 i.e. Riboflavin to the extent of 50 percent of RDA did not reveal any improvement in older adolescent girls after supplementation, yet an improvement to the extent of 8.3 percent of RDA was observed among younger adolescent girls. However, the adequacy of water soluble vitamin B3 i.e. Niacin improved by 39.2 percent and 35 percent of RDA respectively among younger and older adolescents as a result of dietary supplementation. However, no significant change was observed in vitamin A adequacy of both young and old adolescents as a result of dietary supplementation, the deficit being to the extent of 50 percent of RDA (Nanda, 2001).

Besides the quantitative dietary inadequacies, poor quality of dietary protein accounted for growth retardation among these adolescent girls. Diet comprising of vegetable proteins mainly from cereals and pulses and only milk from animal sources constituted the diets of these adolescent girls. A proportion of 5:1 for cereals and pulses has been recommended for best utilization of protein in the diet (Indian Council of Medical Research, 1989). However, disproportionate cereal protein intake resulted in poor utilization of available mixed vegetable protein having Net Protein Utilization (NPU) of 65 percent. In the face of qualitative and quantitative inadequacies of cereal and protein, it could be possible that protein was being utilized for energy purposes and not for growth, thus adversely affecting the growth of these adolescent girls.

Chronic Energy Deficiency (CED) is, thus, the most widespread nutritional deficiency among adolescent girls in the world. It refers to an intake of energy less than the individual requirements for a prolonged period of time. CED is difficult to identify directly because the measurement of energy intake is difficult to obtain. Therefore, CED is usually identified by proxy variables such as deficits in anthropometry, body composition or other growth parameters. There are many researchers who have focused on the problem of CED among Indian populations. Some of them are Ferro-Luzzi et.al. (1992), Khongsdier (2001), Adak et al. (2006), Bharti (1989), Naidu et al. (1991 and 1994), Gautam et al. (2006), Gautam (2007), Gautam and Thakur (2009), Mishra and Mohanty (2009), Gautam et al. (2013), Kumar and Gautam (2015) and Gautam et.al. (2016).

Dietary management should, thus, aims at weight maintenance without compromising on appropriate calorie intake and normal nutrition. Due emphasis should be given to initiate and maintain healthy eating patterns. A standard protocol is to recommend a fat intake of 30 to 40 per cent kcal in children 1 to 3-year-old, with a reduction to 25 to 35 percent in children 4 to 18-year-old; a carbohydrate intake of 45 to 65 percent kcal in all children and adults; and protein intakes of 5 to 20 per cent kcal in children 1 to 3 -year-old with gradual increase to 10 to 30 per cent kcal in children 4 to 18 -year-old (National Academies Press, 2002).

Anthropometric Measurements/ Indices

Physical Anthropologists study human growth with a view to understand constant change, ontogenic conditions and their highly varying tempos at various periods of life (Schultz, 1956). Scientists have been conducting growth studies since the publication of Buffon's work in *Historie Naturelle* in the year 1777. The growth pattern of humans is influenced by several factors, including hereditary and environmental factors.

Growth during adolescence occurs due to rapid accretion of new tissues. Various developmental changes during this phase are accompanied by increased nutritional requirements relative to the nutritional requirements during childhood. When these increased nutritional requirements during adolescence are not met, overall retardation in growth takes place. Height, a linear measurement, is relatively a fixed parameter. It is measurement of skeletal growth and is relatively insensitive to short term nutritional deprivation. However, it is liable to change if nutritional deprivation is of long duration.

The findings of research carried out by the author on anthropometric measurements of adolescent girls of Haryana in India revealed these Indian girls to be shorter and lighter as compared to their respective NCHS standards. The percentile status of these adolescent girls revealed that the deficit in height and weight increased with increasing age. Indices based on height and weight i.e. height-for-age and weight-for-age also revealed the prevalence of stunting to the extent of 31-39 percent and underweight to be 64-68 percent of NCHS standards among these adolescent girls. All circumferential measurements also revealed lower values as compared to their respective standards (Nanda, 2001).

The adolescent girls of the present study revealed a height deficit of great extent which increased with increasing age because the energy demands for other metabolic processes of the body cannot be compromised. Stunting, known to be an index of nutritional status, reflects long term past under-nutrition. Stunting i.e. low height- for-age among these girls could possibly be an outcome of long term calorie and protein deficit in past childhood years, manifesting itself in terms of slowing of their skeletal growth (Nanda, 2001).

When the nutritional deprivation is prolonged, height deficit is also accompanied by weight deficit. Body weight is the most liable parameter and is subjected to alterations within a short period of nutritional manipulations whereas other growth parameters cannot be compromised. So, it is the earliest manifestation of the impact of nutritional manipulations among various anthropometric measurements. Index based on it i.e. weight-for-age is also most liable and is a sure manifestation of continuing past nutritional deprivation of childhood years being reflected in their current nutritional status.

High prevalence of stunting and even higher prevalence of underweight among these adolescent girls suggest that their nutritional deprivation was of long duration, which might have initiated in their childhood years and was continuing during adolescence. Since their dietary intakes during childhood years were not studied, the magnitude of their past nutritional deprivation could not be ascertained in this study (Nanda, 2001).

Correlation analysis between anthropometric measurements/indices and dietary intake of these adolescent girls revealed a highly significantly positive correlation between calories and weight ($r = 0.61$), calories and height ($r = 0.57$), protein and weight ($r = 0.53$) as well as protein and height ($r = 0.49$), indicating that these body measurements were lower in adolescent girls with deficient calorie and protein intake (Nanda, 2001).

The National Nutrition Monitoring Bureau (NNMB) data collected from 10 states of India also showed that the prevalence of stunting was of much higher magnitude to the extent of 50 percent (Sastry, Vijayaraghavan, & Rao, 1989). A UNICEF report also revealed 39 percent prevalence of stunting and 36 percent of underweight among children in developing world (Carlson & Wardlaw, 1990).

A step-wise regression analysis was undertaken to find out the contribution of various factors to the height and weight of these adolescent girls. Results of regression analysis revealed that factors significantly contributing to the weight of these adolescent girls were age, ordinal position, intake of protein, calories, iron, occupation of father and mother, vitamin A and iron intake. Intake of protein, calories, iron and vitamin are known to have significant contribution towards height of these adolescent girls by increasing the muscle mass and mineral skeletal whereas education and occupation of parents reflect the economic status and hence the dietary intake of adolescent girls (Nanda, 2001).

Besides height and weight deficits, nutritional inadequacy was also manifested in terms of lower values of circumferential measurements i.e. Mid Upper Arm Circumference (MUAC), Chest Circumference and Pelvic Girth which also revealed lower values as compared to respective ICMR standards (Nanda, 2001). MUAC is known to reflect changes in muscle tissues and calorie reserves in the form of sub-cutaneous fat. These muscle measurements are the reserves which accumulate only when the calorie and protein intakes are adequate. But in case of huge calorie and protein deficit, it was normal to expect lower values of these circumferential measurements.

The increase in chest circumference during adolescence occurs as a combined result of skeletal growth and fat deposition in connective tissues. The adolescent girls of present study had slightly higher values of chest circumference as compared to respective ICMR standards up to 12 years of age but lagged behind thereafter which is indicative of continued skeletal growth during adolescence but fat deposition would occur only if calorie and protein intakes are adequate (Nanda, 2001).

The pelvic girth measurements are also indicative of skeletal growth and its increase results mainly from changes in pelvic bones. Most, though not all, of the difference in shape of pelvis occurs during adolescence. There exists a close relationship between growth in height and reproductive organ development during adolescence. The correlation between calorie intake and various circumferential measurements was significant, indicating that a reduction in muscle size occurs as a compensation mechanism to provide amino acids for gluconeogenesis and protein synthesis in the liver (Nanda, 2001).

The measurement of skinfold thicknesses in the assessment of nutritional status is based on the assumption that increased subcutaneous fat results from either high calorie intake or low energy expenditure; thus, it reflects a general calorie reserve. Since energy intake was highly deficient in these adolescent girls, lower values of skinfold thicknesses at all the four sites i.e., bicep, tricep, subscapular and suprailliac were an expected outcome in the present study (Nanda, 2001).

When a decrease in thickness of subcutaneous tissues occurs during growth, it does not imply a decrease in cross-sectional area of fat. The fat is a ring around musculoskeletal center which is increasing at all ages. If the cross-sectional area of fat remained constant over the years, during which the muscle and bone core enlarged, then inevitably the fat ring would be stretched thinner. Also, as the fat width diminishes the percentage of body weight due to fat also decreases. While the linear and circumferential measurements are increasing, subcutaneous fat is either shedding or remains unchanged. However, fat deposition increases rapidly as soon as maximum physical dimensions are achieved.

During the period of growth of these adolescent girls, total energy consumed was utilized for somatic growth and an extra energy was required for fat deposition. Lower values of various skinfold thicknesses at all the four sites in these adolescent girls revealed a significant correlation with calorie intake ($r = 0.29$-0.40), indicating that skinfold thicknesses exhibited a reduction in the face of acute energy deficit. A highly significant correlation was found between various skinfold thicknesses and weight ($r = 0.53$-0.77) and BMI ($r = 0.58$-0.73) but less significant with height($r = 0.31$-0.55) (Nanda, 2001). These correlations are suggestive of the fact that only excess energy is stored in adipose tissues after all other requirements of body, including weight gain and BMI are met with. However, height gain continues despite deficit in calorie intake.

The possible responses to inadequate energy intake resulted in retardation in growth in height and weight, loss of fat, loss of muscle, decrease in mass of visceral organs and decrease in basal metabolic rate. The lower values of circumferential measurements and skinfold thicknesses indicating low calorie reserve was perhaps another compensatory mechanism.

Catch-Up Growth

After giving dietary supplementation comprising of cereal-pulse combination along with jaggery for duration of 6 months, a highly significant increase in height and weight of these adolescent girls was observed, thereby resulting in an improvement in the percentile status of adolescent girls of the present research. Height and weight velocities accelerated and the acceleration was higher than the respective NCHS standards, which was indicative of catch-up or compensatory growth as a result of dietary supplementation (Nanda, 2001).

However, it was observed that the acceleration in growth was higher in younger adolescent girls as compared to older adolescent girls because of their growth spurt, which enabled them to catch-up in their growth though not up to the optimum level (Nanda, 2001). The probable reason for higher growth velocities in younger adolescent girls as compared to older adolescent girls could be that the adolescent growth spurt is characterized by rapid gain in lean body mass and even greater increases in adipose tissues along with an increase in mineral skeleton. When the increased nutritional requirements associated with adolescent growth spurt were met, younger adolescent girls gained more height as compared to older adolescent girls. Moreover, younger adolescent girls were in the phase of growth spurt and their nutritional deficit was of shorter duration, hence larger catch-up in growth was observed in contrast to older adolescent girls, who had crossed their growth spurt and had deficit in diet for longer duration, so their catch-up growth was not up to the optimum level.

Among these adolescent girls, height gain was also accompanied by weight gain as a result of dietary supplementation which manifested itself in the form of an increase in adipose tissues, skeletal muscles, bone, blood and visceral organs. Highly accelerated weight velocity i.e. weight gain over a specified period was again indicative of catch-up growth (Nanda, 2001).

However, it was observed that the growth velocities in height were higher than those of weight in all age groups. It is the natural biological phenomenon of the body to continue gain in height, though not to the optimum level, despite a deficit in food intake but gain in weight would occur, only when nutritional needs for somatic growth are met with. Thus, height gain is an earliest response to nutritional intervention followed by weight gain at a minimum genetic potential for height.

Though dietary supplementation improved the nutrient intake of adolescent girls but the increased dietary intake resulted in more improvement in height as compared to weight in view of the alternating priorities of the body for height gain till peak height velocity is attained by these under-nourished adolescent girls because the priorities of the body for muscular and skeletal growth are alternating (Rao & Joshi, 1992).

Higher growth velocities in height among these under-privileged adolescent girls helped them to narrow down but not completely bridge the initial height deficit. Most girls showed catch-up growth regarding height and to some extent regarding weight. The degree of catch-up regarding both height and weight was directly correlated to the degree of under-nutrition (Nanda, 2001).

Linear growth and final height, besides genetic factors, is influenced by nutritional conditions and also by timing of pubertal development, which may be triggered earlier in under-nourished girls undergoing metabolic activation during catch-up growth (Proos, Hofvander, & Tuvemo, 1991). Similar priorities of the body for height gain by under-nourished children and weight gain by normal children have been reported by Rao and Joshi (1992). Studies on the effect of the sudden nutritional improvement showing catch-up growth have also been reported by Marotell et al. (1994).

Another important observation was that the effect of dietary supplementation was greater during nutritional deprivation and is expected to diminish as the nutritional status of adolescent girls improved. It has been reported by Tanner (1990) that catch-up mechanism is based on the fact that catch-up velocity is large to start with and decreases progressively as the target curve is approached. It seems as if the velocity is regulated by a signal of mismatch between the ideal or target curve and the actual situation. Adolescents recover more or less completely by virtue of their regulatory power, provided the adverse conditions are not too long or too severe. In complete catch-up with delay, growth continues for a longer period but in the end, complete catch-up for growth retardation is achieved.

It is a known fact that higher the deficit in food intake, greater is the catch-up growth. There is considerable evidence that significant compensatory or catch-up growth is possible when the growth limiting condition i.e. prolonged under-nutrition is remedied (Largo, 1993). For instance, children who have spent their childhood in poverty and then adopted into affluent families, may show catch-up growth and an early pubertal development, thus reaching the final height in normal range (Proos, 1991).

Proos et al. (1991) studied the menarcheal age and growth pattern of Indian adolescent girls adopted in Sweden and found that most adolescent girls had catch up growth regarding height and half of them regarding weight. The degree of catch up growth regarding both height and weight was directly correlated to the degree of malnutrition. Correlation analysis revealed that adolescent girls with fast catch up and/or late adoption in Sweden had an early menarche. A significant relationship was also found between the menarcheal age and the final height i.e. earlier menarche was associated with shorter final height. The data suggested that linear growth and final height were influenced by the pre-adoptive nutritional conditions.

Indices based on height and weight i.e. height-for-age and weight-for-age are more sensitive indicators of nutritional status. These respond more quickly to variations in nutritional manipulations. Analysis of these indicators also revealed that as a result of intervention, the prevalence of stunting i.e. low height-for-age was reduced by 11 percent and low weight-for-age was reduced by 4 percent among these adolescent girls. Improvement in nutritional status using height-for-age index was highly significant in younger adolescent girls as compared to older adolescent girls, in which it was not significant. It was also observed that adolescent girls, who were severely stunted, improved the most. This was perhaps due to marked increase in lean body mass and mineral skeletal associated with growth spurt in these adolescent girls (Nanda, 2001).

The reduction in the prevalence of stunting by 11 percent and underweight by 4 percent among these adolescent girls suggests that calorie and protein input of dietary supplementation could promote gain in height to some extent, especially in younger adolescent girls who were severely stunted but were not adequate enough to promote weight gain in these adolescent girls. Another possible reason could be priority of the body for height gain by under-nourished adolescent girls. The small reduction in the prevalence of stunting over such a short period was an expected outcome.

Since linear growth is a slow process and even under most favorable conditions takes a relatively long time to show improvement, as also supported by a report of WHO working group (1986). There is good evidence to support that catch-up growth can restore stature of stunted children to normal when nutritional conditions become favorable (Waterlow, 1988).

Gaur and Singh (1994) have also reported a decrease in prevalence of stunting by restoring to normal growth in stature with increasing age through increased hormonal level during adolescence, thus showing catch-up growth. Some cross-sectional studies have also shown that children living in adverse circumstances may experience some catch-up in growth during adolescence without specific intervention (Kulin, H.e., Bwibo, Mutie, & Santner, 1982).

Cameron et al. (1994) have demonstrated that rural children living in impoverished conditions have some capacity to compensate for these circumstances through increased hormonal levels of adolescence combined with increased sensitivity at target sites which allow a more complete expression of the genes dictating adult stature in spite of no major environmental changes.

All the linear measurements of these adolescent girls increased significantly after dietary supplementation, thus indicating skeletal growth during adolescence, until long bones epiphyses fuse which are normally closed by 18 or 19 years of age. However, bones which grow by surface deposition of calcium continue to grow and respond to stimulation even after the growth spurt whereby surface deposition of calcium on these bones occurs due to an increased intake of calcium through dietary supplementation.

All circumferential measurements i.e. chest circumference and pelvic girth of these girls also increased significantly due to growth in bones and flesh as a result of increased number of calories, protein and calcium through dietary supplementation. Significantly positive correlations were found between calorie intake and chest circumference ($r = 0.48$) as well as between calorie intake and pelvic girth ($r = 0.52$), indicating an increase in these circumferences with adequacy of calories in the diet (Nanda, 2001).

Other circumferential measurements i.e. mid upper arm circumference and calf circumference revealed no significant changes because these measurements are known to reflect changes in muscle tissue and calorie reserve in the form of subcutaneous fat and are very sensitive to adequacy of total nutrients. Only excess energy is stored in the adipose tissues of these areas, after all other requirements of the body, including weight gain are met with. No significant change in these measurements was indicative of the fact that increased intake of calories and protein as a result of dietary supplementation was used for somatic growth of these girls and was not adequate enough to be stored as calorie reserve in adipose tissues of these girls. Significantly positive correlations between calorie intake with MUAC (r = 0.50) and between calorie intake with calf circumference (r = 0.48) had been observed which suggest that an increase in MUAC and calf circumference would occur only if calorie intake was adequate enough to meet all other requirements of the body (Nanda, 2001).

Skinfold thicknesses at four sites namely bicep, tricep, subscapular and suprailliac also increased significantly as a result of dietary supplementation, as revealed by significantly positive correlation between dietary intake and skinfold thicknesses at four sites, indicating an increase in various skinfold thicknesses with an increase in calorie intake. With increased calorie intake, adolescent girls were found to have positive energy balance, their energy expenditure being less than their energy intake. Measurement of skinfold thicknesses provides a direct evidence of adequacy or otherwise of calories, independent of the phase of growth spurt.

Significantly positive correlations between skinfold thicknesses and body weight (r = 0.41-0.77), skinfold thicknesses and BMI (r = 0.49-0.72) and less significant in case of skinfold thicknesses with height (r = 0.18-0.59) suggest that adequacy of calories would increase skinfold thicknesses at various sites, after meeting the requirements of body for weight gain and an increase in BMI (Nanda, 2001). However, height gain would occur, though not to the optimum genetic potential, irrespective of the state of adequacy of calories.

Clinical Manifestations

As a consequence of dietary and nutrient inadequacies, several nutritional deficiencies with clinical manifestations were encountered in these adolescent girls, namely protein energy malnutrition (PEM), iron deficiency anaemia (IDA), vitamin deficiencies and iodine deficiency disorder (IDD). Among these nutritional deficiency diseases, anaemia was found to be most prevalent among adolescent girls. Clinical signs of nutritional deficiencies make their appearance, when deprivation has been too long or too severe. It serves as a practical tool for the assessment of nutritional status of the population.

Among various nutritional deficiency diseases prevalent in adolescent girls, the highest prevalence (54.4%) of Iron Deficiency Anaemia was observed, which revealed its manifestation in more than half of girl's population. Pallor of conjunctiva was considered to indicate the deficiency of iron in the body. Results of dietary survey revealed the consumption of cereal based diet, high in phosphorus and phytate content, from which iron absorption is very low (3%). Moreover, highly inadequate consumption of iron and vitamin C along with qualitative and quantitative inadequacy of protein precipitated the symptoms of anaemia in these adolescent girls (Nanda, 2001).

Other nutritional deficiency disease in the descending order of prevalence was Protein Energy Malnutrition (PEM), the incidence being 19.3 percent among these adolescent girls. The qualitative and quantitative inadequacy of good quality protein along with energy deficit resulted in wasteful utilization of protein for energy purposes, thus affecting their health and nutritional status. PEM among these adolescent girls revealed its manifestation in terms of various clinical signs in varying degree of prevalence. The most prevalent signs of PEM were dispigmentation and lack of luster of hair followed by sparseness and easy pluckability of hair. Some of these girls also suffered from muscle wasting and oedema. The sequential appearance of these signs was suggestive of early stages of PEM, which might have precipitated, if the nutritional deficiency continued (Nanda, 2001).

The prevalence of vitamin deficiencies was also found to be high among these adolescent girls. The significantly high prevalence of vitamin C deficiency (15.2%) manifested itself in terms of spongy bleeding gums (12%), recession of gums (10%) followed by petechiae (3%). These were the early signs of vitamin C deficiency manifested due to low intake of vitamin C in their diets. Being a heat sensitive vitamin, fifty percent of vitamin C is lost during cooking, resulting in poor bio-availability of vitamin C to the body (Nanda, 2001).

The deficiency of vitamin B was also significantly high (13.5%) among these adolescent girls. The most commonly found signs of vitamin B deficiency were atrophic papillae, scarlet raw tongue followed by chelosis and angular stomatitis. These were the early signs suggestive of Riboflavin and Niacin deficiency. Dietary intake of these adolescent girls also showed deficient intake of Riboflavin and Niacin to the extent of fifty percent of RDA in their diets.

However, no signs and symptoms of Thiamin deficiency were observed as the intake of Thiamin was found to be adequate in the diet of these adolescent girls. Besides deficient intake of Riboflavin and Niacin, inadequate calorie intake was sure to precipitate the situation because these vitamins serve as co-enzymes for the metabolism and utilization of calories in the body. In the face of acute calorie deficit, if the deficiency of B-vitamins continues, the consequences would be serious (Nanda, 2001).

The prevalence of vitamin D deficiency was 7.6 percent among these adolescent girls which manifested its presence in the form of knock knees and bow legs. Its presence suggested that along with vitamin D availability, low intake of calcium (42-44% of RDA) with its reduced availability due to factors such as phytates in cereal based diets might be responsible for its occurrence in these adolescent girls (Nanda, 2001).

The functional consequences of under-nutrition and anemia found in these adolescent girls resulted in the impairment of their physical work capacity because of reduced oxygen uptake capacity of hemoglobin to carry oxygen to different tissues of the body (Nanda, 2001). The maximum oxygen uptake capacity (an aerobic capacity) is probably the best measure of a person's physical fitness, provided the definition of physical fitness is restricted to the capacity of the individual for prolonged heavy work.

Hematological Profile

The observed deficit in calories, protein, iron and vitamin C, as observed from nutrient intake of these adolescent girls, interfered with the synthesis of haemoglobin. Hematological profile of these adolescent girls also revealed qualitative and a quantitative inadequacy of protein along with deficient intake of iron which interfered with hemoglobin formation, thus resulting in low hemoglobin level of these girls, indicating the incidence of Iron Deficiency Anaemia (IDA) among these adolescent girls. A comparison between the dietary intakes of anaemic adolescent girls and non-anaemic adolescent girls revealed that the dietary intake of calories, protein, iron and vitamin C of non-anaemic adolescent girls was significantly higher than those of anaemic adolescent girls (Nanda, 2001).

Step-wise multiple regression analysis was undertaken to find out the contribution of various factors to the hemoglobin level of these adolescent girls revealed that various significantly contributing factors were age, intake of iron, calcium and vitamin A, occupation of father, education of mother and religion (Nanda, 2001). Intake of iron along with vitamin C and vitamin A have an established role in haemopoises whereas education and occupation of parents indirectly affected the dietary and nutrient intake of these adolescent girls and hence their hematological profile.

It was further observed from the distribution of girls into different grades of anaemia that majority of these adolescent girls were in grade I and II of anaemia. The diet of these girls was rich in phosphorus and phytate content, poor in vitamin C content and had low biological value of protein and consequently low net protein utilization. In a mixed cereal diet, iron is absorbed at the rate of five percent under optimum conditions. Hence, the absorption of iron was bound to be very poor, resulting in poor bio-availability of dietary non-haeme iron, thus precipitating anaemia in these adolescent girls (Nanda, 2001).

Moreover, the older adolescent girls, who had attained menarche at a median age of 11.53 years, had marked losses of iron during menstruation, thus resulting in higher deficit of iron. Hence, with the poor quality and inadequate quantity of diet consumed, coupled with accelerated growth rate and the onset of menarche, the iron balance of these adolescent girls was bound to be negative. This deficit was made good by iron mobilized from tissue stores for hemoglobin synthesis. When the tissue stores were also exhausted, the supply of iron to the marrow for hemoglobin synthesis became inadequate and hypochromic anaemia developed in these girls. In such situations, the red cell count is reduced to a lesser degree than the hemoglobin level and the count may be near normal, even when the haemoglobin level is reduced to 8-9 gm/dl. This was evident from the PCV and RBC levels of these adolescent girls, who were otherwise found to be anaemic (Nanda, 2001).

However, the indices derived from haemoglobin, PCV and RBC i.e. MCV, MCH and MCHC were reduced, the degree of reduction depending upon the severity of anaemia. A subnormal MCV (< approx. 80 fl), MCH (< approx. 27 pg) and MCHC (< approx. 30%) observed in these adolescent girls was indicative of hypochromic microcytic anaemia (Nanda, 2001).

The observed defect in red cell formation could be due to various reasons; one of those could be a condition in which haemoglobin synthesis is impaired to a greater extent, the reason being inadequate iron available for the formation of haeme component of haemoglobin. Hence, subnormal MCV and MCH were indicators of early iron deficient haematopoiesis.

The indicators of iron status among these adolescent girls also revealed a low level of serum iron, a high level of Total Iron Binding Capacity (TIBC) and a low level of transferrin saturation, thereby confirming iron deficiency anaemia in these adolescent girls (Nanda, 2001). The probable reasons could be inadequate intake of iron due to poor diet, diminished bio-availability or impaired absorption and also due to recurrent menstrual losses, thus leading to Iron Deficiency Anaemia in these adolescent girls.

In the development of Iron Deficiency Anaemia, the gradual iron depletion occurs in a sequential manner. In the initial stages of Iron Deficiency Anaemia, the bone marrow stores are utilized to meet the demands of erythropoiesis. During this state of pre-latent iron deficiency, the normal level of storage iron concentration (80 mg %) falls to the level of 29 mg %, the normal TIBC level (290 mg %) rises up to the level of 335-345 mg % but there are no significant changes in haemoglobin level, serum iron and transferrin saturation levels. With further depletion of iron stores, there is inadequate delivery of serum iron to bone marrow for erythropoiesis. TIBC continues to rise while other indicators remain unaffected. This state is known as latent iron deficiency anaemia. Further, TIBC rises up to the level of 380 mg % but there is no overt anaemia. If the iron intake continues to be inadequate, serum iron and transferrin saturation decrease to critical levels. At this level, the formation of haemoglobin is retarded as a result of inefficient erythropoiesis and Iron Deficiency Anaemia or overt anaemia ensues (Weinfeld, 1964).

After giving dietary supplementation along with nutrient supplementation comprising of 20 mg of elemental iron along with 0.1 mg of folic acid for 6 months so as to accrue maximum benefit of dietary supplementation, the haematological profile of these adolescent girls revealed that the haemoglobin level of adolescent girls increased significantly and reached very close to normal level (Nanda, 2001).

Moreover, the distribution of adolescent girls into different grades of anaemia also depicted that majority of the adolescent girls shifted from Grade I and II of anaemia to Normal and Grade I of anaemia. Though there was an improvement in the haemoglobin status of girls in all age groups but the improvement was highly significant in younger adolescent girls (Nanda, 2001). The likely reasons for better response to dietary and nutrient supplementation by younger adolescent girls could be a dramatic increase in lean body mass containing a good deal of iron resulting from increased intake of calories, protein and iron and also an increase in blood volume and haemoglobin, which called for an increase in iron requirement, which was adequately met through dietary and nutrient supplementation and hence these adolescent girls revealed a marked improvement in their haemoglobin level.

However, older adolescent girls, who had entered menarche at a median age of 11.53 years, had marked losses of iron due to mensuration. Despite of this, these adolescent girls improved in their haemoglobin level, indicating that their utilization of iron was good. Despite the availability of adequate amount of iron and other related factors, which enhance iron absorption, the improvement in haemoglobin level, though non-significant, was good enough in the face of losses of iron due to mensuration in the older adolescent girls (Nanda, 2001). Even Benjamin Burton (1978) has reported that the degree of iron absorption depends to a large extent on the current iron balance of the body. This has also been reported by Kapoor and Aneja (1992) and Vasanthi et al. (1994), who have emphasized the need for iron supplementation for adolescent girls, long before they enter puberty.

It was further observed that adolescent girls, who were severely anaemic, improved the most and shifted to higher grades of anaemia. Majority of the adolescent girls from Grade I, II and III improved to Normal, showing a marked improvement in the haemoglobin status of these girls as a result of dietary and nutrient supplementation (Nanda, 2001).

It is a known fact that those, who are severely anaemic, quickly respond to supplementation and improve the most. The height of response to iron supplementation is inversely proportional to the haemoglobin level before supplementation and may exceed normal level in case of severe anaemia. The rate of regeneration is also more marked in early stages and lessens as haemoglobin value approaches normal (de Gruchy, 1990).

Other indicators of haematological profile i.e. PCV and RBC count also increased significantly as a result of dietary and nutrient supplementation and were within the normal range in all age groups. Highly significant correlations have been found between the total dietary intake of iron with haemoglobin (r=0.52), PCV (r=0.61) and RBC (r=0.67), indicating an increase in these haematological indicators with an increase in total iron intake (Nanda, 2001).

The indices i.e. MCV, MCH and MCHC, derived from haemoglobin, PCV and RBC, also improved consequent upon the dietary and nutrient supplementation. The indicators of iron status in the body i.e. serum iron, TIBC and transferrin saturation were also found to undergo significant positive changes in all age groups of adolescent girls (Nanda, 2001).

Serum iron, bound to a specific protein, transferrin, is kinetically the most active compartment of total iron in the body because it is normally replaced and recycled at least ten times daily. Its value increased significantly and was within the normal range. With the increase in serum iron level, TIBC, which is the capacity of serum protein transferrin to bind 2.5-4.0 mg of iron/ litre, decreased significantly in all age groups and was within the normal range after supplementation, indicating better availability of iron for haemoglobin synthesis. Thus, with increased serum iron level, the formation of haemoglobin was improved as a result of efficient erythropoiesis and overt anaemia was corrected (Nanda, 2001).

National Institute of Nutrition (NIN) in Hyderabad conducted a Nutrition Surveys in the selected states of India during the years from 2001 to 2006. Data revealed that more than half of the adolescent population, aged 10-18 years, was undernourished (NNMB, 2002; NNMB, 2006).

NNMB Surveys were carried out in the year 2001 in the states of Andhra Pradesh, Gujarat, Karnataka, Kerala, Madhya Pradesh, Maharashtra, Orissa, Tamil Nadu and West Bengal. Results of the survey revealed that 78 per cent of the surveyed population in 10 to13 years age group and 66 per cent of the surveyed population in 14 to17 years age group were observed to be undernourished. Micronutrient deficiencies ranged from 1 to 2 per cent in these populations.

NNMB Surveys carried out in the year 2006 among the rural populations of Kerala, Karnataka, Tamil Nadu, Andhra Pradesh, Maharashtra, Madhya Pradesh, Gujarat, Orissa and West Bengal revealed that out of 51,700 populations, of which 5530 adolescents, aged 12 to17 years, selected by two stage stratified random sampling technique, were covered for dietary information. Nutrition assessment was done using anthropometry (compared with NCHS standards), clinical examination along with the dietary survey. Prevalence of under nutrition was found to be 38 percent in both 10 to13 years and 14 to17 years age groups and micronutrient deficiencies ranged from 1 to 3 percent in these populations.

Rao et al. (2003) carried out a community-based study in rural areas of Kundam blocks of Jabalpur in Madhya Pradesh, India. For this study, a sample of 818 adolescent boys and girls, aged 11 to 19 years, were selected by probability proportional to size sampling technique. Nutritional status was assessed using NCHS reference data with anthropometric measurements taken by using standardized techniques. Findings of the study revealed that 61.7 percent adolescents were underweight and 51.7 percent were stunted. Wasting was observed in 32.8 percent of adolescents. In adolescent boys and girls, prevalence rate of anaemia was 82.3 percent of the surveyed population.

A cross-sectional community-based study was undertaken on 270 rural adolescent girls by Choudhary et al. (2003) in Chiraiga block of Varanasi in Uttar Pradesh, India. Sample for the study was selected by simple random sampling technique. Nutritional status was assessed by weight-for-age, height-for-age, weight-for-height, MUAC-for-age and BMI at different age points. Results of this study revealed that 68.52 percent adolescent girls were underweight (BMI < 18.5 kg/m2). It was also found that 19.63 percent adolescent girls suffered from CED Grade-I; corresponding values for Grade-II and Grade-III were 17.78 and 31.11 percent respectively. Micronutrient deficiencies ranged from 3 to 25 percent among the selected population.

A community based cross-sectional study was conducted by Deshmukh et al. (2006) in Wardha district in the state of Maharashtra in India. In the rural areas, 764 adolescents were selected by two stage sampling method. Nutritional status was classified using mean BMI-for-age with CDC (2000) reference standards. It was found that 53.8 percent of the adolescents were thin, 75.3 percent of them had Chronic Energy Deficiency (CED) and 20.8 percent of adolescents suffered from wasting.

Haboubi et al. (2009) carried out a cross-sectional survey in Kerala, Tamil Nadu and UAE among school based 2459 adolescent boys and girls, aged 10 and 16 years (1200 from Kerala and Tamil Nadu in India and 1259 from UAE). Adolescents were found to be falling below the age and gender-specific 5th and 3rd percentiles of the WHO recommended standards. India specific data showed that 38.8 percent of boys and 36.9 percent girls were stunted and 64.6 percent boys and 50.1 percent girls were thin.

A national level study carried out by Parsuraman et al. (2009) on 47,590 women and 24,997 men, aged 15-24 years, selected by multi-stage stratified sampling technique using Structured Questionnaire revealed that 44 percent women and 47 percent men, aged 15-24 years, were abnormally thin. It was also found that 56 percent of women and 25 percent of men were anaemic among rural populations.

Maliye et al. (2010) conducted a cross-sectional study in the rural areas of Sewagram, Wardha where 430 unmarried adolescent girls, aged 10-19 years, were assessed with the help of pre-designed and pre-tested questionnaire; CDC 2000 reference standard was used to assess the nutritional status of adolescent girls. Findings of this study revealed that 57 percent of the adolescent girls were thin and undernourished.

A cross-sectional study was undertaken by Wasnik et al. (2012) in urban areas of Vizianagaram, Andhra Pradesh covering 420 adolescent girls, aged 10 to 15 years, using predesigned, pretested, semi-structured schedule. Anthropometric measurements were recorded using standardized methodology as recommended by WHO. Results of the study revealed that 56.4 percent of adolescent girls were undernourished. Among those undernourished adolescent girls, 25.2, 15.2 and 16 percent were suffering from Chronic

Energy Deficiency (CED) grade I, II and III, respectively and 30 percent of them were found to be anaemic.

Sahani and Das (2015) carried out a survey on the growth pattern of Ahom adolescents from Sibsagar, Assam to study their growth and development pattern during adolescent period and to see the sexual difference in the pattern of their growth. The study concentrated on growth pattern of adolescents from 11 to 17 years of age from different ethnic groups and ecological zones. The results of the study indicated that the Ahom adolescents were shorter and lighter than the NCHS reference data and Beijing reference data but taller than the Rabhas, Moplah, Kaibarta and others. It could, thus, be concluded that the growth pattern of Ahom adolescents was in general satisfactory.

All other variables considered in this study carried out by Sahani and Das (2015) on the growth pattern of Ahom adolescents from Sibsagar, Assam showed a constant increase among the present Ahom boys and girls. However, the triceps skinfold measurements in boys showed a variable trend. The sex differences were significant in bi-acromial diameter, triceps skinfold, BMI, calf circumference and chest circumference measurements. The comparison of the present data with that of 1976 data of the same population did not give any clear-cut idea, probably due to different sampling cluster. However, in comparisons to the data from Sonowal Kachari of the same year, the present Ahom boys were taller, except at 12 and 13 years of age. Ahom girls were taller than Sonowal Kachari girls.

Most of the variables considered in this study showed more mean values in Ahom boys than the Sonowal Kachari boys. But in case of girls, the comparison was not so distinct. Similarly, the present Ahom boys and girls showed a comparatively more mean values of stature and weight and other variables than the Khasi adolescents (Khongsdier & Mukherjee, 2003a; 2003b) and Assamese Muslim and Rabhas adolescents. In comparison with Moplah of Andaman, the Ahom adolescents were always ahead, except the skin fold measurements at triceps.

Most of the variables considered in this work showed a spurt at 13 years of age in both sexes. However, a few measurements and indices, such as MUAC, triceps skin fold, BMI and cormic index measurements in boys did not show spurt at 13 years of age but showed it later at 14, 15 and 16 years respectively. In case of girls, only cormic index did not show spurt at 13 years of age while remaining measurements and indices showed a spurt at 13 years.

In another study, Sahani et al. (2018) conducted a cross-sectional analysis of anthropometric data of 2010 individuals of 19 different groups of indigenous islanders of Andaman and Nicobar Islands. The data was collected by the trained anthropologists of Anthropological Survey of India by following standard techniques and ethical guidelines. It was found that the indigenous islanders have small body size as compared to immigrants and their counterparts. The prevalence of chronic energy deficiency (CED) was found highest among the mainlanders. Highest prevalence of overweight was found among Great Andamanese (18.2%), followed by Onge (7.4%). Individuals below 21 years of age were not found to be overweight or obese. On the other side, 16.7 percent of individual of age 41 years and above of local born were found to be overweight (BMI 25.0-29.9 kg/m2). It can be concluded that the indigenous people of the Islands were short in stature and nutritionally better than immigrants. The immigrants were better than their counterparts in the mainland but still they were not able to reach at par of the indigenous people in the level of nutrition.

Findings of the above studies lead one to conclude that poor nutritional status of adolescents is an outcome of socio-cultural, economic and public policies relating to household food security compounded by behavioural dimensions. These undernourished and anemic adolescent girls/mothers are at a high risk of miscarriage, maternal mortality and still births; also, low birth weight babies with low iron reserves that, in turn, grow into vulnerable adults and are burden on the society.

Overweight and Obesity

Conversely, overweight and obesity – another form of malnutrition with serious health consequences is increasing among other young people in India and other Low Middle Income Countries (LMICs) (World Health Organization, 2011).

Worldwide, disease profiles are transforming at a rapid pace catching the attention of medical professionals and policy makers alike. This is particularly true in low and middle-income countries that form the major chunk of global population. The emerging epidemics of obesity, cardiovascular disease (CVD) and diabetes form the crux of this phenomenal change. Among these entities, obesity has become a colossal epidemic causing serious public health concern and contributes to 2.6 million deaths worldwide every year (WHO, 2005).

Obesity is associated with an increased risk of morbidity and mortality as well as reduced life expectancy. The last two decades of the previous century have witnessed dramatic increase in health care costs due to obesity and related issues among children and adolescents (Wang & Dietz, 2002).

Childhood obesity affects both developed and developing countries of all socio-economic groups, irrespective of age, sex or ethnicity. It has been estimated that worldwide over 22 million children under the age of 5 years are obese, and one in 10 children is overweight (Kosti & Panagiotakos, 2006).

A wide range of prevalence levels exist, with the prevalence of overweight in Africa and Asia averaging well below 10 percent and in the Americas and Europe above 20 percent. The proportion of school-age children affected has almost doubled by 2010 as compared with the available surveys from the late 1990s up to 2003 (Kosti & Panagiotakos, 2006).

Obesity has become a serious public health concern affecting a significant portion of the population in countries like United States of America. Overall, among adults aged at least 20 years in years 1999-2002, 65.1 percent were overweight, and 30.4 percent were obese. Among children, aged 6 through 19 years, during 1999-2002, 31.0 percent were overweight, and 16.0 percent were obese (Hedley, Ogden, Johnson, Carroll, Curtin, & Flegal, 2004).

However, the Asian countries are not immune to this phenomenon. For example, in China, the prevalence of overweight and obesity among children, aged 7-9 years, increased from 1 - 2 percent in 1985 to 17 percent among girls and 25 percent among boys in the year 2000 (Wang, Kong, Wu, Bai, & Burton, 2005).

In addition, obesity prevalence varies across socio-economic strata. In developed countries, children of low socioeconomic status are more affected than their affluent counterparts (Strauss & Pollack, 2001). The opposite is observed in developing countries i.e. children of the upper socio-economic strata are more likely to be obese than poor children (Salmon, 2005; Chhatwal, 2004).

Similar socio-economic trends in childhood obesity in India are also emerging. A study from northern India reported a childhood obesity prevalence of 5.59 percent in the higher socio-economic strata when compared to 0.42 percent in the lower socio-economic strata (Marwaha, 2006).

Indian data regarding current trends in childhood obesity are emerging. A recent study conducted among 24,000 school children in south India showed that the proportion of overweight children increased from 4.94 percent of the total students in 2003 to 6.57 percent in 2005, thereby demonstrating the time trend of this rapidly growing epidemic (Raj, Sundaram, Paul, Deepa, & Kumar, 2007).

In addition to growth deficits among indigenous populations (Agrahar-Murugkar, 2005; Mitra, Kumar, Ghosh, & Bharati, 2002; Reddy & Rao, 2000), growth excesses in the form of overweight and obesity are also increasingly reported in India in many studies (Kabir, 2005; Pandher, Sangha, & Chawla, 2004; Sharma, 2002). It may be due to the fact that the country has become industrialized and undergone a rapid nutritional transition (Kapoor & Anand, 2002; Shetty, 2002) similar to that of other low-income countries (Popkin, 1994; Popkin, Richards, & Montiero, 1996). Therefore, in developing countries such as India, childhood obesity for the last few decades have also become an important health issue (Bouchard, 2000; Cole, Bellizzi, Flegal, & Dietz, 2000).

Obesity can be assessed throughout childhood growth years which are a good measure of health and nutritional status of a population, particularly in children because it is sensitive to variation in the environmental quality (Frisancho, 1990; Khongsdier, 1999; Waterlow, Buzina, Keller, Lane, Nichama, & Tanner, 1977).

For children and adolescents, overweight and obesity are defined using age and sex specific normograms for body mass index (BMI). Children with BMI equal to or exceeding the age-gender-specific 95th percentile is defined obese. Those with BMI equal to or exceeding the 85th but are below 95th percentiles are defined overweight and are at risk for obesity related co-morbidities (Donohoue, 2004).

Khongsdier and Mukherjee (2003) have rightly pointed out that an improvement in socio-economic status, better nutrition and access to health amenities were likely to be more important factors for better growth and development among children. Longitudinal studies from childhood to adulthood have shown that overweight children may become overweight adults if obesity persists in adolescence (Mo-suwan, Tongkumchum, & Peutpaiboon, 1998).

In that respect, Sahani (2004) and Sahani et al. (2010) have observed that increase in obesity is a recent emerging phenomenon among Nicobarese adults in Nicobar Islands of India. It may be due to change of their lifestyle and food habits. In order to find out whether childhood obesity or trend towards obesity also persists among Nicobarese children of Car Nicobar Island, specifically among a pre-adolescent group, an attempt to assess the growth and nutritional status among Car Nicobarese children using anthropometric indices was made. These results were compared with results for children of Moplah community of Andaman Island who lived in a similar environment as children from Car Nicobar Island.

For this comparison, Sahani et al. (2014) carried out a cross-sectional study to assess the growth and nutritional status of Car Nicobarese children and compared it with Moplah children, who lived in a similar environment. A total of 436 Car Nicobarese children and 438 Moplah children, aged 6–10 years, were selected for this study. The anthropometric measurements included stature, body weight, sitting height, bi-acromial breadth, bi-iliac breadth, mid-upper arm circumference, skinfold thickness of biceps, triceps and subscapular region. The 50th percentile (median) growth curves were calculated among the studied children and compared with Centers for Disease Control and Prevention (CDC) 2000 reference standards. The Z scores of weight-for-age (WAZ), height-for-age (HAZ) and BMI-for-age (BMIZ) were computed using growth references of the CDC (2000). It was observed that the Car Nicobarese children were shorter but heavier than Moplah children of both sexes all through the age range which was also reflected in the median values of anthropometric variables. Car Nicobarese children were nutritionally better as compared to Moplah children based on the nutritional indices. The major differences between Car Nicobarese and Moplah children were found in their arm muscularity rather than arm adiposity. Overall, Car Nicobarese children were nutritionally in normal and better condition than Moplah children. However, present dietary change (intake of high calories and fat diet) of Car Nicobarese population may be reflected in the form of childhood obesity which has already been observed in their adult population.

Another study carried out by Sahani (2013) on the anthropometry and nutrition of Onges of Little Andaman Island examined the impact of forced settlement among the foraging Onges which induced them to change their subsistence from full time foragers to settled consumers. In this experimental study, anthropometric along with dietary investigations were considered before and afterwards they were forcibly settled. The anthropometric variables and indices showed a gradual increase among the Onges males but not so much in females. High prevalence of overweight and obesity was also reported. Comparison with other Andaman Islanders indicated that the group which was under the developmental schemes (forced to settle) was showing more mean values of anthropometric variables with prevalence of overweight and obesity than the group which was not under the influence of developmental program. Their dietary pattern and physical activity changed to a great extent. The protein content of the diets reduced significantly and the fat along with carbohydrates increased to a substantial amount. The contribution of protein to calories has been reduced substantially and now it is only around 10 percent whereas in the past it was above 30 percent. Caloric intake increased more than two times while the physical activity level reduced to about half time. Decreased mobility and altered food habits could be the probable reasons for the gradual increase of body dimensions and prevalent overweight and obesity which were the outcomes of forced settlement.

A meta-analysis of various studies childhood and adolescent overweight and obesity carried out during the years 2001 to 2012 showed 12.6 percent of children to be overweight and 3.3 percent to be obese, indicating the seriousness of the situation.

Meta-analysis of nine studies in India among 67,919 children for obesity and 92,862 children for overweight was carried out by Midha et al. (2012). Children and adolescents, aged 2 to 19 years, were selected in these studies. CDC/WHO criteria for classification of obesity were used. Prevalence of overweight and obesity was found to be 12.64 and 3.39 percent respectively. The overall prevalence rate was 12.64 percent among these children and adolescents.

NNMB (2001) carried out various surveys among rural populations of Andhra Pradesh, Gujarat, Karnataka, Kerala, Madhya Pradesh, Maharashtra, Orissa, Tamil Nadu and West Bengal in India, in which 51,239 adolescents was covered for assessment. Sample for the surveys was selected by two-stage stratified random sampling method. Nutrition assessment was done using anthropometry, clinical examination and dietary survey. Prevalence of obesity was found to be 0.6 percent among rural adolescents.

Khadilkar et al. (2004) conducted an urban school based cross-sectional study on 1228 boys, aged 10 to 15 years, from Pune, Maharashtra in India who were selected by stratified random sampling technique. The international criteria for Body Mass Index were used for classifying children as overweight and obese. Indian standards for 85th and 95th percentile was adapted. Prevalence of overweight was 19.9 percent and obesity were 5.7 percent among this population.

Laxmaiah et al. (2007) conducted a school based cross-sectional study in urban area of Hyderabad, Andhra Pradesh in India, for which 1150 adolescents, aged 12 to 17 years, were selected by multistage stratified cluster sampling technique. Overweight and obesity assessment was defined by the IOTF criteria. Prevalence of overweight was found to be 6.1 percent among boys and 8.2 percent among girls; Obesity prevalence was found to be 1.6 and 1.0 percent among boys and girls respectively.

Kumar et al. (2007) undertook an urban school based cross-sectional study in Davangere, Karnataka in India which was followed by case control study among 1496 school children, aged 10 to 15 years. Calculation of Body Mass Index was based on KN Agarwal percentiles. Overall prevalence of obesity was found to be 5.74 percent with rates of 4.4 percent among boys and 8.8 percent among girls.

Mehta et al. (2007) carried out an urban school based cross-sectional study on 414 adolescent girls, aged 16 to 17 years, from Delhi in India. Sample was selected by random sampling method. For the assessment of nutritional status of adolescent girls, BMI > 30 kg/m2 (i.e. > 95th percentile) denotes obesity and BMI > 25 kg/m2 (i.e. > 85th percentile) denotes overweight, according to IOTF criteria. Using this criterion, the prevalence of overweight among adolescent girls was 15.2 percent and obesity was 5.3 percent amongst these adolescent girls.

Aggarwal et al. (2008) conducted a school based cross-sectional study representing affluent schools in urban area of Ludhiana, Punjab in India. For this study, a sample of 1000 adolescents was selected by random and purposive sampling technique. Pre-validated questionnaire was used for data collection. Nutritional status assessment was done using anthropometry with international cut-off points for the Body Mass Index; BMI > 95th percentile for age and sex were considered as obese and BMI >85th percentile was considered as overweight. Prevalence of overweight among boys and girls was 15 and 10.2 percent respectively and overall prevalence of obesity was found to be 3.4 percent among these adolescents.

Kotian et al. (2010) undertook a school-based cross-sectional study in urban area of Mangalore, Karnataka in India. A sample of 900 adolescents, aged 12 to 15 years, was selected by multistage stratified random sampling technique. Questionnaire and anthropometric measurements were used for assessment of the nutritional status. Prevalence of overweight and obesity was found to be 9.9 percent and 4.8 percent respectively.

Goyal et al. (2011) carried out a cross-sectional study among urban adolescents from two private schools in Surat city, Gujarat in India. A sample of 1209 adolescents, aged 12 to 15 years, was selected by simple random sampling method. Pre-designed and pre-tested questionnaire was used along with weight measurement using Growth Monitoring Guidelines recommended by IAP. Overall prevalence of overweight and obesity was 13.9 percent and 6.55 percent respectively. However, the prevalence of overweight and obesity among boys was found to be 15.1 percent and 6.7 percent respectively and among girls, the prevalence was 13.35 percent and 6.4 percent respectively.

Another study by Sikandra et al. (2014) was carried out among 400 obese school children, aged 9 to15 years, who were selected randomly from Hisar and Gurugram city in Haryana, India. Hundred healthy school children of same age having no history of obesity were taken as control group. Information on Socio-economic status (SES), food habits and dietary pattern was gathered using self-developed questionnaire. Results of the study revealed that the prevalence of obesity was higher (7.41%) among children from Gurugram as compared to children from Hisar (5.79%). It was found that playing outdoor games was the main activity of non-obese children (36%). Majority of obese children (78%) were not doing any physical activity and only 7 percent of obese were doing cycling and 13 percent were doing walking as their exercises. It was noticed that more than 50 percent of obese children spent less than 6 hours for sleeping.

It is clear from the meta-analysis of above studies that India is facing the dual burden of under-nutrition on one side and over-nutrition on the other, as also seen from other reports (Jeemon, 2009; Srihari, 2007). There is also a challenge of nutritional transition as Indians are moving away from traditional diets high in cereal and fiber to more western pattern diets high in sugars, fat and animal-source food (fast food culture) that are closely associated with different non-communicable diseases (NCD's) seen in later years (Mohan, 2007; Shetty, 2002).

Analyzing the probable reasons for nutritional transition among adolescents, the use of mass media was found to be higher among adolescents (male 88.2 percent and female 71.5 percent) (UNICEF, 2013). Mass media plays an important role in habit picking and decides their lifestyle pattern. Its influence is clearly shown in a study from Chennai in India, conducted on adolescents in the age group of 11 to 17 years which reported that 90 percent of adolescents ate either food or snacks while watching television, 82 percent bought food products and snacks based on advertisement, 59 percent skipped outdoor activities for watching television, 42 percent followed junk diet and 42 percent exercised to get their body like their favorite media personality (Priyadarshini, 2013). Television viewing during childhood and adolescence is associated with overweight, poor fitness, smoking and raised cholesterol level in adulthood (Hancox, 2004).

Adolescents have increased nutritional requirements demanding diet rich in protein, vitamins, calcium, iodine, phosphorus and iron due to rapid growth spurt and increased physical activity. NFHS-3 data shows, in the age group 15 to19 years, 47 percent girls and 58 percent boys were thin, 56 percent girls and 30 percent boys were anemic, 2.4 percent girls and 31.7 percent boys were overweight and 2/1000 adolescent girls and 1/1000 adolescent boys suffer from diabetes. They are also highly prone for eating disorders like anorexia nervosa or binge eating disorders due to body dissatisfaction and depression (Sivagurunathan, UmaDevi, Rama, & Gopalakrishnan, 2015).

Iron Deficiency Anaemia (IDA) is the leading cause of Years Lost to Death and Disability among female adolescents during the year 2015. Iron and folic acid supplements is a solution that also helps to promote health before adolescents become mothers. Regular deworming in areas where intestinal helminths such as hookworm are common is recommended to prevent micronutrient (including iron) deficiencies (Sivagurunathan, UmaDevi, Rama, & Gopalakrishnan, 2015).

The treatment of overweight and obesity in children and adolescents requires a multidisciplinary approach with a holistic outlook. The team should include a paediatric physician, nurse practitioner, dietician, physical instructor, behavioural therapist and a social worker in addition to a motivated team of parents, caretakers, teachers and policy makers. The immediate goal is to bring down the rate of weight gain, followed by a period of weight maintenance and finally weight reduction to improve Body Mass Index. The long-term goal is to improve quality of life and reduction in morbidity as well as mortality associated with overweight and obesity (Raj & Krishna Kumar, 2010).

Exercise and Nutrition

In the light of findings of the above studies on overweight and obesity, it can be inferred that increased energy intakes and decreased protein consumption is one of the causes of the prevalent overweight and obesity. In addition, the decreasing physical activity level (PAL) and higher energy intake may play a role in the existing overweight and obesity levels. The decrease of PAL, in spite of the decline in energy intakes, is associated with the increase of obesity already reported in the UK (Prentice & Jebb, 1995). Social ecological theory also suggests that individual's health is determined by multiple levels of influence including institutional level, community, broader physical, economic and cultural environmental factors (McLeroy, Bibeau, Sleckler, & Glanz, 1988).

Developing healthy eating and exercise habits during adolescence are foundations for good health in adulthood. Reducing the marketing of foods high in saturated fats, trans-fatty acids, free sugars or salt, providing access to healthy foods and opportunities to engage in physical activity are important for good health of all, especially for children and adolescents. Yet available survey data indicates that 1 in every 4 adolescents meets the recommended guidelines for physical activity: 60 minutes of moderate to vigorous physical activity daily.

Other Infectious Diseases

Thanks to improved childhood vaccination, adolescent deaths and disability from Measles have fallen down markedly by 90 percent in the African Region between the years 2000 and 2012. However, Diarrhoea and Lower Respiratory Tract Infections (LRTI's) are estimated to be among the top five causes of deaths for 10 to 19-year-old adolescents. These two diseases, together with Meningitis, are the top three causes of adolescent deaths in African Low and Middle-Income Countries (LMIC's).

In India, data on adolescents from national surveys including National Family Health Survey III (NFHS-3), District Level Household Survey and Facility Survey III and Sample Registration System calls for a focused attention with respect to health and social development for this age group. It has, therefore, been realized that investing in adolescent health will yield demographic and economic dividends for India.

In view of this, Government of India launched its first comprehensive program for adolescents, 'Rashtriya Kishor Swasthya Karyakram' during January 2014 which has a sharp focus on adolescents physical and reproductive health. The program envisages that all adolescents in India are able to realize their full potential by making informed and responsible decisions related to their health and well-being (Ministry of Health and Family Welfare, 2014).

Thus, supplementary feeding program, as envisaged in adolescent health programs of Government of India, is of paramount importance for promoting catch-up growth in undernourished adolescent girls, if given regularly in judicious combination and at a higher quantum for a longer duration. Moreover, supplementary feeding is of proven benefit for promoting optimum catch-up growth in adolescent girls, especially in the period of growth spurt i.e. at least 18 to 24 months prior to menarche. Adolescent growth spurt offers an opportunity to adolescent girls to make up for the growth retardation of the past childhood years. It can help to narrow down, though not completely, and bridge the initial growth retardation.

Besides, many health policies and programs initiated by the government have focused on prioritized individual health problems but integrated (both vertical and horizontal) coordinated approaches are found lacking. Healthy life-style and health promotion policies and programs that are central for health of youth, driven by robust population-based studies are required in India which will also address the growing tide of NCD's and injuries.

Thus, the ultimate goal is to identify strategies that can foster service integration and coordination across public and private health systems so that the two sectors can complement each other in addressing the health needs of today's adolescents, strengthen adolescent's capacity to become healthy and productive adults and ultimately achieve the objectives of healthy adolescents for healthy nation.

REFERENCES

ACC/SCN. (1991). *Controlling Iron Deficiency*. Nutrition Policy Discussion Paper No. 9, 22.

Adak, D. K., Gautam, R. K., & Gharami, A. K. (2006). Assessment of Nutritional status through Body Mass Index among adult males of 7 tribal populations of Maharashtra, India. *Malaysian Journal of Nutrition, 12*(1), 23–31.

Aggarwal, T., Bhatia, R., Singh, D., & Sobti, P. C. (2008). Prevalence of obesity and overweight in affluent adolescents from Ludhiana, Punjab. *Indian Pediatrics, 45*, 500–502. PMID:18599939

Agostoni, C., Rottoli, A., Trojan, S., & Riva, E. (1994). Dairy products and adolescent nutrition. *The Journal of International Medical Research, 22*(2), 67–76. doi:10.1177/030006059402200201 PMID:8020640

Agrahar-Murugkar, D. (2005). Nutritional status of Khasi schoolgirls in Meghalaya. *Nutrition (Burbank, Los Angeles County, Calif.), 21*(4), 425–431. doi:10.1016/j.nut.2004.07.012 PMID:15811761

Benjamin Burton, T. (1978). Human Nutrition (3rd ed.). Academic Press.

Bharati, P. (1989). Variation in adult body dimensions in relation to economic condition among the Mahishyas of Howrah district, West Bengal, India. *Annals of Human Biology, 16*(6), 529–541. doi:10.1080/03014468900000662 PMID:2589818

Bouchard, C. (2000). The obesity epidemic: introduction. In C. Bouchard (Ed.), *Physical Activity and Obesity* (pp. 3–20). Champaign, IL: Human Kinetics Publishers.

Cameron, N., Gordon-larsen, P., & Wrchote, E. M. (1994). Longitudinal analysis of adolescent growth growth in height, fitness and fat patterning in rural South African black children. *American Journal of Physical Anthropology, 93*(3), 307–321. doi:10.1002/ajpa.1330930304 PMID:8042694

Carlson, B. A., & Wardlaw, T. M. (1990). *A global, regional and country assessment of child malnutrition*. UNICEF staff working paper No. 7. UNICEF.

Chhatwal, J., Verma, M., & Riar, S. K. (2004). Obesity among pre-adolescent and adolescents of a developing country [India]. *Asia Pacific Journal of Clinical Nutrition, 13*, 231–235. PMID:15331333

Choudhary, S., Mishra, C. P., & Shukla, K. P. (2003). Nutritional status of adolescent girls in rural area of Varanasi. *Indian Journal of Preventive and Social Medicine*, *34*, 53–61.

Cole, T. H., Bellizzi, M. C., Flegal, K. M., & Dietz, W. H. (2000). Establishing a standard de.nition for childhood overweight and obesity worldwide: International survey. *British Medical Journal*, *320*(7244), 1240–1243. doi:10.1136/bmj.320.7244.1240 PMID:10797032

Datta, B. (1982). Semi longitudinal growth evaluation of childrenfrom birth to 14 years in different socio-economic groups. *Indian Pediatrics*, *19*, 353–359. PMID:7141647

deGruchy. (1990). *Clinical Haematology in Medical Practice*. Oxford Medical Press.

Deshmukh, P. R., Gupta, S. S., Bharambe, M. S., Dongre, A. R., Maliye, C., Kaur, S., & Garg, B. S. (2006). Nutritional status of adolescents in rural Wardha. *Indian Journal of Pediatrics*, *73*(2), 139–141. doi:10.1007/BF02820204 PMID:16514223

Donohoue, P. A. (2004). Obesity. In R. E. Behrman, R. M. Kleigman, & H. B. Jenson (Eds.), *Nelson Textbook of Pediatrics* (17th ed.; pp. 173–177). Philadelphia: WB Saundersp.

Ferro-Luzzi, A., Sette, S., Franklin, M., & James, W. P. T. (1992). A Simplified approach of assessing adult chronic energy deficiency. *European Journal of Clinical Nutrition*, *46*, 173–186. PMID:1559522

Forbes, G. B. (1980). *Nutritional requirement in adolescents in Suskind, R.B. Paediatric Nutrition*. New York: Raven Press.

Friedman, H. L. (1994). Adolescent health care, International Initiatives. *Indian Pediatrics*, *31*, 503–510. PMID:7875880

Frisancho, A. R. (1990). *Anthropometric Standards for Assessment of Growth and Nutritional Status*. The University of Michigan Press. doi:10.3998/mpub.12198

Gaur, R., & Singh, N. Y. (1994). Nutritional status among ural Meitei children of Manipur, India. *American Journal of Human Biology*, *6*(6), 731–740. doi:10.1002/ajhb.1310060607 PMID:28548324

Gautam, R. K., Adak, D. K., & Bharati, P. (2016). Extent of Chronic Energy Deficiency among Central Indian Tribes. In N. Mondal & J. B. R. Sen (Eds.), *Nutrition and health among Tribal population of India* (pp. 231–239). Delhi: Publishing Corporation.

Gautam, R, K., Adak, D.K., Gharami, A.K., & Datta, T. (2006). Body mass index in Central India: inter-district variation. *Anthropologischer Anzeigrer*, 447-61.

Gautam, R. K., Adak, D. K., Pal, M., & Bharati, P. (2013). Morphometric variation among the Central Indian populations. *Human Biology Review*, *2*(2), 153–175.

Gautam, R. K., Adak, D. K., Pal, M., & Bharati, P. (2013). Morphmetric variation among the central India populations. *Human Biology Review*, *2*(2), 153–175.

Gautam, R. K., & Thakur, R. (2009). Biosocial correlate of nutrition and chronic energy deficiency among adult females of two ecological zones in Madhya Pradesh and Uttarakhand, India. *Malaysian Journal of Nutrition*, *15*(2), 137–153. PMID:22691812

Goyal, J. P., Kumar, N., Parma, I., Shah, V. B., & Patel, B. (2011). Determinants of overweight and obesity in affluent adolescent in Surat city, South Gujarat region, India. *Indian Journal of Community Medicine*, *36*(4), 296–300. doi:10.4103/0970-0218.91418 PMID:22279261

Haboubi, G. J., & Shaikh, R. B. (2009). A comparison of the nutritional 20. status of adolescents from selected schools of South India and UAE: A cross-sectional study. *Indian Journal of Community Medicine*, *34*(2), 108–111. doi:10.4103/0970-0218.51230 PMID:19966955

Hancox, R., Milne, B., & Poulton, R. (2004). Association between child and adolescent television viewing and adult health: A longitudinal birth cohort study. *Lancet*, *364*(9430), 257–262. doi:10.1016/S0140-6736(04)16675-0 PMID:15262103

Hedley, A. A., Ogden, C. L., Johnson, C. L., Carroll, M. D., Curtin, L. R., & Flegal, K. M. (2004). Prevalence of overweight and obesity among US children, adolescents, and adults 1999-2002. *Journal of the American Medical Association*, *291*(23), 2847–2850. doi:10.1001/jama.291.23.2847 PMID:15199035

Indian Council of Medical Research. (1989). *Nutritive Value of Indian Foods*. Hyderabad, India: National Institute of Nutrition.

Jeemon, P., Prabhakaran, D., Mohan, V., Thankappan, K. R., Joshi, P. P., & Ahmed, F. (2009). Double burden of underweight and overweight among children (10-19 years of age) of employees working in Indian industrial units. *The National Medical Journal of India*, *22*, 172–176. PMID:20131480

Kabir, Z. (2005). Adult chronic disease and childhood obesity: A life course approach in developing countries? *International Journal of Epidemiology*, *34*(2), 481–482. doi:10.1093/ije/dyi017 PMID:15737972

Kapoor, G., & Aneja, S. (1992). Nutritional disorders in adolescent girls. *Indian Pediatrics*, *29*(8), 969–973. PMID:1459717

Kapoor, S. K., & Anand, K. (2002). Nutrition transition: A public health challenge in developing countries. *Journal of Epidemiology and Community Health*, *56*(11), 804–805. doi:10.1136/jech.56.11.804 PMID:12388563

Khadilkar, V. V., & Khadilkar, A. V. (2004). Prevalence of obesity in affluent school boys in Pune. *Indian Pediatrics*, *41*, 857–858. PMID:15347879

Khongsdier, R. (2001). Body mass index of adult males in 12 populations of Northeast India. *Annals of Human Biology*, *28*(4), 374–383. doi:10.1080/03014460010004610 PMID:11459235

Khongsdier, R., & Mukherjee, N. (2003). Growth and nutritional status of Khasi boys in Northeast India relating to exogamous marriages and socioeconomic classes. *American Journal of Physical Anthropology*, *122*(2), 162–170. doi:10.1002/ajpa.10305 PMID:12949836

Khongsdier, R., & Mukherjee, N. (2003a). Growth and nutritional status of Khasi boys in Northeast India relating to exogamous marriages and socioeconomic classes. *American Journal of Physical Anthropology*, *122*(2), 162–170. doi:10.1002/ajpa.10305 PMID:12949836

Khongsdier, R., & Mukherjee, N. (2003b). Effects of heterosis on growth in height and its segments: A cross-sectional study of the Khasi girls in Northeast India. *Annals of Human Biology*, *30*(5), 605–621. doi:10.1080/0301446031 0001592669 PMID:12959901

Kosti, R. I., & Panagiotakos, D. B. (2006). The epidemic of obesity in children and adolescents in the world. *Central European Journal of Public Health*, *14*(4), 151–159. doi:10.21101/cejph.a3398 PMID:17243492

Kotian, M. S., Kumar, S. G., & Kotian, S. S. (2010). Prevalence and determinants of overweight and obesity among adolescent school children of South Karnataka, India. *Indian Journal of Community Medicine*, *35*(1), 176–178. doi:10.4103/0970-0218.62587 PMID:20606948

Kulin, H., Bwibo, N., Mutie, D., & Santner, S. J. (1982). The effect of chronic childhood malnutrition on pubertal growth and development. *The American Journal of Clinical Nutrition*, *36*(3), 527–536. doi:10.1093/ajcn/36.3.527 PMID:7113957

Kumar, A., & Gautam, R. K. (2015). Obesity and chronic deficiency among adult bidi workers of Central India. *International Journal of Interdisciplinary and Multidisciplinary Studies*, *2*(5), 60–69.

Kumar, S., Mahabalaraju, D. K., & Anuroopa, M. S. (2007). Prevalence of obesity and its influencing factor among affluent school children of Davangere city. *Indian Journal of Community Medicine*, *32*(1), 15–17. doi:10.4103/0970-0218.53384

Largo, R. H. (1993). Catch-up growth during adolescence. *Hormone Research*, *39*(Suppl. 3), 41–48. doi:10.1159/000182783 PMID:8262491

Laxmaiah, A., Nagalla, B., Vijayaraghavan, K., & Nair, M. (2007). Factors affecting prevalence of overweight among 12- to 17-year-old urban adolescents in Hyderabad, India. *Obesity (Silver Spring, Md.)*, *15*(6), 1384–1390. doi:10.1038/oby.2007.165 PMID:17557974

Malina, R. M., & Bouchard, C. (1991). *Growth, Maturation and Physical Activity*. Human Kinetics Book.

Maliye, C., Deshmukh, P., Gupta, S., Kaur, S., Mehendale, A., & Garg, B. (2010). Nutrient intake amongst rural adolescent girls of Wardha. *Indian Journal of Community Medicine*, *35*(3), 400–402. doi:10.4103/0970-0218.69264 PMID:21031105

Marotell, R., Kettel Khan, L., & Schroeder, D. G. (1994). Reversibility of stunting: Epidemological findingsin children from developed countries. *European Journal of Clinical Nutrition*, *48*(Suppl. 1), S45–S57.

Marwaha, R. K., Tandon, N., Singh, Y., Aggarwal, R., Grewal, K., & Mani, K. (2006). A study of growth parameters and prevalence of overweight and obesity in school children from Delhi. *Indian Pediatrics*, *43*, 943–952. PMID:17151397

McLeroy, K. R., Bibeau, D., Sleckler, A., & Glanz, K. (1988). An ecological perspective on health promotion programs. *Health Education & Behavior, 15*, 351–377. PMID:3068205

Mehta, M., Bhasin, S. K., Agrawal, K., & Dwivedi, S. (2007). Obesity amongst affluent adolescent girls. *Indian Journal of Pediatrics, 74*(7), 619–622. doi:10.100712098-007-0109-8 PMID:17699967

Midha, T., Nath, B., Kumari, R., Rao, Y. K., & Pandey, U. (2012). Childhood obesity in India: A meta-analysis. *Indian Journal of Pediatrics, 79*(7), 945–948. doi:10.100712098-011-0587-6 PMID:22002317

Mishra, B. K., & Mohanty, S. (2009). Dietary intake and nutritional anthropometry of the workers of INDAL, Hirakud. *Anthropologist, 11*(2), 99–107. doi:10.1080/09720073.2009.11891089

Mitra, M., Kumar, P. V., Ghosh, R., & Bharati, P. (2002). Growth pattern of the Kamars – a primitive tribe of Chhattisgarh, *India. Collegium Antropologicum, 26*, 485–499. PMID:12528272

Mo-suwan, L., Tongkumchum, P., & Peutpaiboon, A. (1998). Determinants of overweight tracking from childhood to adolescent: A 5 years follow up study based on the Boyd Orr cohort. *The American Journal of Clinical Nutrition, 67*, 1111–1118. doi:10.1093/ajcn/67.6.1111 PMID:9625081

Mohan, V., Sandeep, S., Deepa, R., Shah, B., & Varghese, C. (2007). Epidemiology of type 2 diabetes: Indian scenario. *The Indian Journal of Medical Research, 125*, 217–230. PMID:17496352

Naidu, A. N. (1994). Body mass index: A measure of the nutritional status in Indian population. *European Journal of Clinical Nutrition, 48*(3), S131–S140. PMID:7843150

Nanda, S. (2001). *Assessment of an Improved module of National Adolescent Girls Scheme and Evaluation of the Ongoing Scheme* (Unpublished doctoral dissertation). Panjab University, Chandigarh, India.

National Academies Press. (2002). Dietary reference intakes for energy, carbohydrate, fiber, fat, fatty acids, cholesterol, protein, and amino acids (macronutrients). Washington, DC: Author.

National Institute of Nutrition. (1998). *Dietary Guidelines for Indians- A Manual*. Hyderabad: Indian Council of Medical Research.

National Nutrition Monitoring Bureau. (2002). *Diet and nutritional status of rural population.* Hyderabad: National Institute of Nutrition; p. 158. NNMB Technical Report No. 21. Available from: http://www.nnmbindia.org/NNMBREPORT2001-web.pdf

National Nutrition Monitoring Bureau. (2006). *Diet & nutritional status of population and prevalence of hypertension among adults in rural areas.* Hyderabad: National Institute of Nutrition. Available from: http://www.nnmbindia.org/NNMBReport06Nov20.pdf

National Research Council. (1989). *Recommended Dietary Allowances* (10th ed.). Washington, DC: National Academy Press.

Pandher, A. K., Sangha, J., & Chawla, P. (2004). Childhood obesity among Punjabi children in relation to physical activity and their blood profile. *Journal of Human Ecology (Delhi, India), 15*(3), 179–182. doi:10.1080/09709274.2004.11905688

Parsuraman, S., Kishor, S., Singh, S. K., & Vaidehi, Y. (2009). *A profile of youth in India. National Family Health Survey (NFHS-3), India, 2005-06. Mumbai: International Institute for Population Sciences.* Calverton, MD: ICF Macro. Available from http://www.rchiips.org/NFHS/youth_report_for_website_18sep09.pdf

Popkin, B. M. (1994). The nutrition transition in low income countries: An emerging crisis. *Nutrition Reviews, 52*(9), 285–298. doi:10.1111/j.1753-4887.1994.tb01460.x PMID:7984344

Popkin, B. M., Richards, M. K., & Montiero, C. A. (1996). Stunting is associated with overweight in children of four nations that are undergoing the nutrition transition. *The Journal of Nutrition, 126*(12), 3009–3016. doi:10.1093/jn/126.12.3009 PMID:9001368

Prentice, A. M., & Jebb, S. A. (1995). Obesity in Britain: Gluttony or sloth? *British Medical Journal, 311*(7002), 437–439. doi:10.1136/bmj.311.7002.437 PMID:7640595

Priyadarshini, R., Jasmine, S., Valarmathi, S., Kalpana, S., & Parameswari, S. (2013). Impact of media on the physical health of urban school children of age group 11-17 yrs in Chennai – A cross sectional study. *IOSR Journal of Humanities and Social Science, 9*(5), 30–35. doi:10.9790/0837-0953035

Proos, L. A., Hofvander, Y., & Tuvemo, T. (1991). Menarcheal age and growth pattern of Indian girls adopted in Sweden, II catch-up growth and final height. *Indian Journal of Pediatrics*, *58*(1), 105–114. doi:10.1007/BF02810420 PMID:1937614

Raj, M., & Krishna Kumar, R. (2010). Obesity in children and adolescents. *The Indian Journal of Medical Research*, *132*, 598–607. PMID:21150012

Raj, M., Sundaram, K. R., Paul, M., Deepa, A. S., & Kumar, R. K. (2007). Obesity in Indian children: Time trends and relationship with hypertension. *The National Medical Journal of India*, *20*, 288–293. PMID:18335794

Rao, S., & Joshi, S. (1992). importance of periodic measurements in evaluating feeding programmes. *The Indian Journal of Medical Research*, *96*, 45–52. PMID:1597331

Rao, V. G., Aggrawal, M. C., Yadav, R., Das, S. K., Sahare, L. K., & Bondley, M. K. (2003). Intestinal parasitic infections, anaemia and undernutrition among tribal adolescents of Madhya Pradesh. *Indian Journal of Community Medicine*, *28*, 26–29.

Rashtriya Kishor Swasthya Karyakram and National Consultation on Adolescent Health. (2014). Ministry of Health and Family Welfare. Available from: http://rksklaunch.in/rkskl-strategy.html

Reddy, P. Y. B., & Rao, A. P. (2000). Growth pattern of the Sugalis – a tribal population of Andhra Pradesh, India. *Annals of Human Biology*, *27*(1), 67–81. doi:10.1080/030144600282398 PMID:10673142

Regmi, S. C., & Adhikari, R. (1994). *A study of factors influencing nutritional status of adolescent girls in Nepal*. Washington, DC: International Centre for Research for Women.

Sahani, R. (2003). Nutritional and health status of the Jarawas: A preliminary report. *Journal of the Anthropological Survey of India*, *52*, 47–65.

Sahani, R. (2004). Seasonal variation in the nutritional status of the Jarawas. *Journal of the Anthropological Survey of India*, *53*, 99–116.

Sahani, R. (2013). Foraging to settled life: A comparative study of anthropometry and nutrition of Onges of Little Andaman Island. *HOMO - Journal of Comparative Human Biology*, *64*, 391–397.

Sahani, R., & Das, B. (2015). Growth Pattern of Adolescent Ahom Children from Sibsagar, Assam. *Indian Journal of Physical Anthropology and Human Genetics*, *34*(1), 57–69.

Sahani, R., Gautam, R. K., Goldani, A. H., & Vedwan, N. (2018). Comparative study of chronic energy deficiency among adult males of Andaman and Nicobar Islands and their counterparts. *Anthropological Review*, *81*(1), 1–18. doi:10.2478/anre-2018-0001

Salmon, J., Timperio, A., Cleland, V., & Venn, A. (2005). Trends in children's physical activity and weight status in high and low socioeconomic status areas of Melbourne, Victoria, 1985-2001. *Australian and New Zealand Journal of Public Health*, *29*(4), 337–342. doi:10.1111/j.1467-842X.2005.tb00204.x PMID:16222931

Sastry, J. G., Vijayaraghavan, K., & Rao, N. P. (1989). Indian preschool children- A profile of stunting and wasting. *Journal of Tropical Pediatrics*, *35*(5), 237–240. doi:10.1093/tropej/35.5.237 PMID:2511334

Schultz, A. V. (1956). Post embryonic age changes. *Primatologia*, *1*, 887.

Senapati, S. K., Bhattacharya, S., & Das, D. K. (1990). The girl child: An exposition of their status. *Indian Journal of Community Medicine*, *1*, 15–19.

Sharma, M. (2002, March 3). Roly Poly Children Make Unfit Adults. *The Tribune (Spectrum)*.

Shetty, P. S. (2002). Nutrition transition in India. *Public Health Nutrition*, *5*(1a), 175–182. doi:10.1079/PHN2001291 PMID:12027282

Sikandra, R. & Kumar, V. (n.d.). *Prevalence of obesity among school going adolescents*. Developmental Prospects of Life Sills. Women Studies and Development Cell, Haryana.

Singh, S., & Gururaj, G. (2014). Health behaviours & problems among young people in India: Cause for concern & call for action. *The Indian Journal of Medical Research*, *140*, 185–208. PMID:25297351

Sivagurunathan, C., UmaDevi, R., Rama, R., & Gopalakrishnan, S. (2015). Adolescent Health: Present Status and Its Related Programmes in India. Are We in the Right Direction? *Journal of Clinical and Diagnostic Research*, *9*(3), 1-6.

Srihari, G., Eilander, A., Muthayya, S., Kurpad, A. V., & Seshadri, S. (2007). Nutritional status of affluent Indian school children: What and how much do we know? *Indian Pediatrics*, *44*, 204–213. PMID:17413196

Stang, J., & Story, M. (2005). Guidelines for Adolescent Nutrition Services.. University of Minnesota.

Strauss, R. S., & Pollack, H. A. (2001). Epidemic increase in childhood overweight, 1986-1998. *Journal of the American Medical Association*, *286*(22), 2845–2848. doi:10.1001/jama.286.22.2845 PMID:11735760

Tanner, J. M. (1962). *Growth at Adolescence* (2nd ed.). Blackwell.

Tanner, J. M. (1990). *Foetus into man: Physical growth from conception to maturity*. Cambridge, MA: Harvard University Press.

Unicef. (2013). *Statistics Adolescents*. Retrieved September 8, 2014 from http://www.unicef.org/infobycountry/india_statistics.html

Vasanthi, G., Pawashe, A. B., Susie, H., Sujatha, T., & Raman, L. (1994). Iron nutritional status of adolescent girls from rural area and urban slum. *Indian Pediatrics*, *31*, 127–132. PMID:7875834

Wang, G., & Dietz, W. H. (2002). Economic burden of obesity in youths aged 6 to 17 years: 1979-1999. *Pediatrics*, *109*(5), E81–E1. doi:10.1542/peds.109.5.e81 PMID:11986487

Wang, L., Kong, L., Wu, F., Bai, Y., & Burton, R. (2005). Preventing chronic diseases in China. *Lancet*, *366*(9499), 1821–1824. doi:10.1016/S0140-6736(05)67344-8 PMID:16298221

Wasnik, V., Rao, B. S., & Rao, D. (2012). A study of the health status of early adolescent girls residing in social welfare hostels in Vizianagaram district of Andhra Pradesh state, India. *International Journal of Collaborative Research on Internal Medicine and Public Health*. Available from: http://iomcworld.com/ijcrimph/ijcrimph-v04-n01-07.htm

Waterloo, J. C. (1988). Observations on the natural history of stunting. In Linear growth retardation in less developed countries. New York: Vevey/Raven Press.

Waterlow, J. C., Buzina, R., Keller, W., Lane, J. M., Nichama, M. Z., & Tanner, J. M. (1977). The presentation and use of height and weight data for comparing the nutritional status of children under ten years. *Bulletin of the World Health Organization*, *55*, 489–498. PMID:304391

Weiner, J. S., & Lourie, J. A. (1981). *Practical Human Biology*. London: Academic Press.

Winfield, A. (1964). Storage iron in man. *Acta Medica Scandinavica. Supplementum*, 427. PMID:14222360

World Health Organization. (2005). Preventing chronic diseases: Avital investment. World Global Report. Geneva: WHO.

World Health Organization. (2011). *Young people: health risks and solutions. Fact sheet no. 345*. *8*. Available from: http://www.who.int/mediacentre/factsheets/fs345/en/index.html

Chapter 3
Psycho-Social Health

ABSTRACT

Adolescence is the period when development is less gradual and more salutatory, suggestive of some ancient period of storm and stress when old moorings were broken and higher level attained. Important functions previously non-existent arise. Every step of the upward way is strewn with wreckage of body, mind, and morals. It is inherently a time when all young people go through some degree of emotional and behavioral upheaval before establishing a more stable equilibrium in adulthood. Interest in adult life and in vocations develops. Youth awakes to a new world and understands neither it nor him. Character and personality are taking form, but everything is plastic. Self-feelings and ambitions are increased, and every trait and faculty is pliable to exaggeration and excess. Both cognitive and behavioral processes affect them, thus affecting the psycho-social health of adolescents.

KEY FACTS

- Estimated 1.2 million adolescents died in the year 2015, nearly over 3000 every day, mostly from preventable or treatable causes.
- Road traffic injuries were the leading cause of death in the year 2015.
- Other major causes of adolescent deaths included lower respiratory tract infections, suicides, diarrhoeal diseases and drowning.
- Half of all mental health disorders in adulthood start by the age of 14 years but most cases usually remain undetected and untreated. (Adolescent Health World Document)

DOI: 10.4018/978-1-5225-7384-5.ch003

INTRODUCTION

Adolescence is a critical developmental period with long-term implications for the health and well-being of the individual and for society as a whole. The most significant factors to adolescents' health are found in their environments and in the choices and opportunities for health-enhancing or health-compromising behaviors that these contexts present (e.g., exposure to violence, supportive families etc.). Inadequate contexts represent a failure to invest in and protect adolescents, a choice to alienate rather than integrate them into society.

Adolescents form a socially important segment of the population. However, there is no organized system to govern and monitor the social needs of adolescents which contributes towards their holistic health and wellbeing. The Committee on the Gopalakrishnan Rights of the Child (CRC, WHO) published its guidelines in 2013 on the rights of children and adolescents and issued guidelines on states obligations to recognize the special health and developmental needs and rights of adolescents and young people. This has been further envisaged in WHO report in 2014, titled "Health for the World's Adolescents".

Adolescence is a psycho-physical and psycho-social period during which most adolescents adjust to radical changes in their bodies, outgrow the psychological response of childhood and begin to acquire behavior which most adults use with varying degree of sources; as a transition or link between childhood and adult stage. An adolescent is exposed to a number of risk factors like increased sexual desire and no outlet, peer pressure, aggression, victimization, bullying, alcoholism, depression, suicide thoughts etc.

This chapter focuses on the magnitude psycho-social health issues and concerns of adolescents along with strategies to improve mental health status of adolescents as well as the challenges involved so as to create awareness among adolescents and the stakeholders about the importance of strengthening the adolescent health care services so as to meet their felt needs for holistic health and well-being.

Psycho-Social Health

Human beings are highly influenced by both psychological and social factors. It is the interaction between these two forces that determines how the individual will cope up in the world. Psychological and social problems, particularly involving human behavior and responses, are more common during adolescence than at any other time in the life of an individual. During this phase, adjustment to the changing psycho-social environment makes them mature and responsible adults. If adequate care and attention is not given, adolescents are likely to develop various psycho-social problems with long standing impact on their wellbeing and that of the society.

Traditionally, adolescence has been considered as a period stress and storm resulting from glandular and other changes. An adolescent comes under social pressures and faces new conditions for which he received little training during childhood. At this stage, adolescent begins to worry about his future when he realizes that his schooling has come to an end. Gasell and others (1956) observed that adolescents are often irritable, are easily excited and explode emotionally instead of trying to control their feelings. In this way, stress and storm of this period lessens as early adolescence draws to a close.

Elizabeth B. Hurlock (1976) describes the emotional state of the adolescent as …'being treated like a child' or 'being treated unfairly' which is more likely to make the adolescent angry than anything else. Instead of having temper tantrums, however, the adolescent expresses his anger by being sulky, refusing to speak or loudly criticizing those who anger him. The adolescents also become envois of those whose material possessions are superior to him.

In Psychology and its Bearing on Education, C.W. Valentine (1957) gave results of 200 confidential essays on adolescents. According to him, the main sources of mental trouble to the adolescents were of intense self-consciousness resulting from extreme awkwardness, strong feelings of inferiority, unhappy relations with parents, doubts about religion, disgust or fear at the first experience of sexual emotion or of pre-mature advances and at times distress social evils which seem insolvable unless the individual could have a free hand to deal with them.

In the words of Richmond,

The restlessness, the changing mood, the flaming enthusiasm, often short lived, the romantic fantasies and the tendency of day dreaming, the self-conceit and self-assertion characteristics arise from the deepest recesses of their nature. Adolescence is the heyday of the emotional life, the blossom time of all those feelings and emotions which depend at the bottom upon sex.

For generations in India, families remained as supportive and nurturing units providing survival, security, affiliation, love and care to its members.

Most of the children in the world are born in an environment of concern and care for its children, adolescents, parents and grandparents for the fulfillment of their psycho-social needs. The breakdown of traditional families and now the nuclear and single parent families have created social isolation and loneliness and starved children and adolescents of emotional support, thus resulting in various psycho-social problems.

Psycho-Social Needs of Adolescents

Adolescents have various special needs to be fulfilled for their psycho-social well-being (Aggarwal, 2014):

- **Need for Autonomy:** Young adolescents need freedom in their lives. They do not like to maintain a strict routine life. They do not like a disciplined life which is imposed on them by their parents. They love taking independent decisions related to various aspects of their lives leading to autonomy and hence empowerment.
- **Need for Security:** Adolescents seek love and affection, care and concern as well as attention of their parents for the satisfaction of their security needs. Parents become their role models with whom they identify themselves, worship and derive strength and inspiration, imbibe values and character, help formulate life goals and ambitions to shape their personality.
- **Adventure Needs:** Thirst for adventure is strong at this age. Adolescents want to do something novel and innovative so that there are remembered by all for exploring new and different things. In this process, they are often misunderstood and misinterpreted. In the lack of guidance, it often becomes aimless wandering, vagabonding and sometimes indulging in anti-social activities. Sometimes, they also indulge in sexual activities for thrill and adventure.
- **Need for Self-Dependence:** Adolescents want to be independent and begin to think seriously about their future. They become seriously concerned about their occupation with greater security and less demand on their time.
- **Need for a Vocation**: They are concerned about what they would like to do and what they are capable of doing. As a result of greater realism, they approach the choice of their careers with more practical and more realistic attitude.

- **Need for Social Life**: Adolescents want the company of peers and want to live with their peers who have direct influence on their lives. They want to talk, discuss with them and come to some conclusion which goes a long way towards satisfying their social needs. They want approval of their actions and recognition in any form by their parents, peers, teachers and community at large.

Achieving Identity: A Key Task of Adolescence

Erik Erikson (1968), in his developmental theory, elaborated that the adolescents undergo dilemma between role identity and role conflict. Seeking identity involves searching for continuity in oneself and trying to get a clear sense of one's skills and the personal attributes are to discover where one is headed in life and that one can count on recognition from significant others.

According to Erikson (1968), Adolescents who form a sense of identity gain two benefits which are," A feeling of being at home in one's body" and "A sense of psychological wellbeing." He also speaks of Psychological Moratorium i.e. an adolescent may delay in taking up responsibilities and rebellion pattern wherein adolescents go against their parents and well-wishers in spite of being told for their own good.

In confusion and identity crisis, adolescents try to understand their strengths and weaknesses. He seeks to establish his identity in the world around. Confusion sets in when he is not sure of his potentialities and skills, he has to hone up his skills and set them in tune to his personality. He needs to identify his role in the society and strive towards that goal. Once he is focused towards his goal, he has vision to reach and the confusion ends.

In the present century, urbanization and industrialization has pushed children and adolescents down the priority list of parents in both developing as well as developed countries. According to a study in Britain by Abbey National, four out of ten Britons have too little time to spend with the people who mean the most to them. More than a third is so busy that they have forgotten a loved one's birthday or anniversary. Two third of parents admit that they are unable to cope with the housework and nearly half of the parents confess that they cannot reconcile the demands of careers and the needs of their children and adolescents. This scenario has emerged as a general trend all over the world.

The sufferers of this trend are innocent children and adolescents. Presently, millions of young children and adolescents are homeless or shelter less and their number has almost doubled in last two decades. In United States of

America, a homeless girl in her early teens is 14 times more vulnerable to pregnancy than a girl within a home.

In such a scenario, adolescents become vulnerable to emotional stress because of rapid physical, sexual, psychological and social transition. Physically, stress occurs due to sexual maturation and other secondary physical changes that occur during puberty and results in hormonal changes. As a child nears puberty, a gland in the brain, called pituitary gland, increases the secretion of a hormone, Follicle Stimulating Hormone (FSH). This hormone causes additional effects. In girls, FSH activates the ovaries to start producing estrogen. In boys, it causes sperms to develop. The role of good nutrition for the growth of adolescents needs to be considered which otherwise results in poor physical health and nutritional status.

These biological changes affect the adolescents, both internally as well as externally. Internally, the body undergoes hormonal changes. At this crucial phase, the lack of counseling and advice by the parents and teachers could stem the deviant behavior. It can cause disorders and it may even precipitate to suicide and an adrenaline rush often leads to risky behavior. The internal imbalance may also result in extreme emotional behavior that could harm an adolescent.

The external factors like parent's divorce, domestic violence, bad company and unhealthy habits would affect adolescent's psychology, where they experience deviant behavior due to lack of parental attention and extreme indulgence.

Psychologically, stress is an outcome of or an individual's response to a stimulus as a result of an interaction of the person with his/her environment; physical, psychological or social, that creates stress to which the individual responds in a manner which depends on several intrinsic and/or extrinsic factors. Significant difficulties have been experienced in quantifying and qualifying stress among adolescents.

Social change is also a crucial stressor as it is the phase when adolescents prefer to spend time outside the home and demand for freedom. In a relationship between adolescents and their parents, the central theme is often that of testing limits. In this phase, parents can expect less obedience and more resistance that is because adolescents can think of alternatives to parent's rules. Thus, the relationship between parents and adolescents is vital during these disturbed times. The emotional support which the parents give is very essential as this would keep them in constant touch with their parents and would be easy to take care of them. In the absence of such a parent child relationship, adolescent would try to seek emotional support outside the family which could be dangerous.

A study conducted on adolescents by Cassey (2010) indicates that adolescence is a period of stress and storm. In spite of intense and frequent negative effects, this period has been hypothesized to explain increased rates of affective disorders, suicides and accidental deaths. Yet some emerge from adolescence with minimal turmoil. The environmental factors may exacerbate the turmoil of adolescents.

Challenges

However, adolescents are confronted with many challenges throughout the world. Denial of opportunities and recognition to girls and women is widespread in almost all parts of the world. Their contributions, achievements and sacrifices often go unnoticed and unrecognized. Occupational segregation around the world has kept majority of women outside economic, professional and political avenues. Despite great advancements, girls around the world continue to live in an unequal and impoverished environment.

All over the world, the age of marriage is rising, and the age of menarche has been falling. Teenage pregnancy is on the rise in many developing countries. Young adolescents are caught in a vortex between changing values and attitudes of traditional and transitional societies. Therefore, parents, teachers and planners have to be more responsive to the physical, psychological, social and vocational needs of adolescents, who are the real resource of the country.

The new century should provide such role models for adolescents that make safer behavior more attractive. Their reproductive health needs require attention on top priority. Every year 15 million adolescents less than 20 years of age give births which account for one fifth of all births worldwide.

Youth development programs must take into account by designing youth friendly program. Radical changes in attitude and behavior of adolescents need to be understood. This requires inter-generational communication and dialogue. Peer education models are becoming popular and more effective. Both young and old need to change their mutual perception for a harmonious transition to new ways of living without sacrificing their roots and positive values.

Psycho-Social Dysfunction

It has been well understood that adolescence is the transitional stage of development between childhood and adulthood, representing the period of time during which a person experiences a variety of biological and emotional changes. Hall has described this phase as a "Period of Storm and Stress" and remarked that "conflict at this developmental stage is normal" (Hall, 1904).

Ahmad et al. (2007) has explained the internalizing and externalizing disorders among adolescents, the most common psycho-social dysfunctions during adolescence being depression and anxiety (internalizing disorders), delinquency, aggression, educational difficulties and truancy (externalizing disorders).

Globally, 1 out of 5 (20%) adolescents encounter at least one or the other behavioral problem. Half of life time mental disorders begin before the age of 14 years and 75 percent of mental disorders begin by the age of 24 years (World Health Organization, 2001, Kessler, Berglund, Demler, Jin, Merikangas, & Walters, 2005). Studies carried out in Canada and USA have shown that mental health problems among the adolescent population is a public health issue (Jellinek, Murphy, Little, Pagano, Comer, & Kelleher, 1999; Polaha, Dalton, & Allen, 2011).

In developing countries such as Nepal and other South-Asian countries, scenario of mental health problems and its care system is worse as compared to developed countries. In the Indian context, 14 to 40 percent of adolescent students are assumed to have mental health problems (Ahmad, Khalique, Khan, & Amir, 2007; Muzammil, Kishore, & Semwal, 2009; Arumugam, Rajendran, & Nagalingam, 2013).

Lack of attention to the mental wellbeing of children and adolescents, in a key phase of socialization, may lead to mental health consequences that may remain throughout life and reduce the capacity of societies' socio-economic productivity (World Health Organization, 2001; Wittchen, Nelson, & Lachner, 1998).

Thus, it can be concluded that psycho-social development of adolescents is an outcome of their physical, psychological, social and emotional well-being which, in turn, is reflected in their satisfactory academic performance. This ultimately contributes to reduce the risk of psycho-social and behavioral problems, violence, crime, teenage pregnancy and misuse of drugs and alcohol

(Keyes, 2007; NICE, 2008; NICE, 2009; NICE, 2010). Identification and early detection of psycho-social dysfunction during early adolescence helps in improving their quality of life as an adult.

Adolescent's well-being is mainly affected by the home and school environments. Besides home as an institution of social development, school plays a significant role in the overall educational and socialization processes which are crucial for the personality development of an adolescent (Greenbaum, 1974).

However, mental health problems are one of the most neglected issues among adolescents. Mortality and morbidity due to mental disorders among adolescents has increased manifold and have topped in the recent years. A study from Goa, among 16 to 24 years old population, shows that 3.9 percent of youth reported suicidal behavior, with females four times more prone than males. This suicidal behaviour is independently associated with factors like absenteeism, independent decision making, premarital sex, sexual abuse, physical abuse from parents and mental disorders (Pillai, 2009).

Other behavioral issues include substance use disorders (tobacco, alcohol and others), Road Traffic Injuries (RTI's), suicides (completed or attempted), Sexually Transmitted Infections (STI's) including Human Immuno-deficiency Virus (HIV) infection, teen and unplanned pregnancies, homelessness, violence and several others. In all countries, whether developing, transitional or developed, disabilities, acute and chronic illnesses are often induced or compounded by economic hardship, unemployment, sanctions, restrictions, poverty or poorly/ unevenly distributed wealth at both individual and country level (World Youth Report, 2003).

Multiple behavioural disorders and conditions often co-exist in the same individual, thus adding a cumulative risk for their poor health and longevity. Many of these conditions are precursors and determinants of non-communicable diseases (NCD's), including mental and neurological disorders and injuries which place a heavy burden on any society in terms of mortality, morbidity, disability and socio-economic losses (Singh & Gururaj, 2014).

In India, suicide rate among adolescents is higher than in any other age groups to the extent that 40 percent of suicide deaths in men and 56 percent of suicide deaths in women occurred in 15 to 29 years of age group (Patel, 2012). The prevalence rate of child and adolescent psychiatric disorders in the community has been found to be 6.46 percent and in schools, it was 23.33 percent. Moreover, the reporting systems of psychiatric disorders in children are found to be inadequate (Malhotra & Patra, 2014; Rani & Karunanidhi,

2010). From the above studies, it is evident that a considerable proportion of adolescents have mental health problems.

Common Mental Disorders

Around 20 per cent of adolescents around the world are likely to suffer from mental illnesses such as depression, mood disturbances, substance abuse, suicidal behaviours, eating disorders and others (World Health Organization, 2011). A meta-analysis of five psychiatric epidemiological studies yielded an estimated prevalence of mental morbidity including 16 mental and behavioural disorders (classified into eight groups of organic psychosis, schizophrenia, manic affective psychosis, manic depression, endogenous depression, mental retardation, epilepsy, phobia, generalized anxiety, neurotic depression, obsession and compulsion, hysteria, alcohol/drug addiction, somatisation, personality disorders and behavioural/emotional disorders) to the extent of 22.2 per 1000 population among 15 to 24 years old population (Reddy & Chandrashekar, 1998).

Research findings indicate a high incidence of mental disorders among adolescents in India. The morbidity rate due to psychiatric disorders (depression, conduct disorder, social anxiety, panic disorder) among this population has ranged from 12 to 16.5 percent (Srinath, 2005; Anita, 2003).

Among the few specific common mental disorders, the incidence of depression has ranged from 0.1 to 18.5 percent (Srinath, 2005; Anita, 2003; Nair, Paul, & John, 2004; Ahmad, Khalique, Khan, & Amir, 2007; Bansal, Goyal, & Srivastava, 2009; Sahoo & Khess, 2010), conduct disorders from 0.2 to 9.2 percent (Srinath, 2005; Anita, 2003; Ahmad, Khalique, Khan, & Amir, 2007) and anxiety from 0.1 to 24.4 percent (Srinath, 2005; Anita, 2003; Pillai, Patel, Cardozo, Goodman, Weiss, & Andrew, 2008; Ahmad, Khalique, Khan, & Amir, 2007; Sahoo & Khess, 2010; Deb, Chatterjee, & Walsh, 2010) across different studies.

Two studies were undertaken by Nair et al. (2004) and Bansal et al. (2009) which assessed the incidence of severe and extreme grade of depression using Beck's Depression Inventory. Findings of these studies revealed that 11.2 percent of the school dropouts, 3 percent of the school going adolescents, aged 13 to 19 years and 18.4 percent of the 9th standard students suffered from severe and extreme grade of depression.

A community-based study was conducted by Anita et al. (2003) among 800 children, aged 6 to 14 years, in urban and rural areas of Rohtak, Haryana in India. The subjects were assessed for psychiatric symptoms, using CPMS and diagnostic assessment using DISC. Results revealed that 16.5 percent of children, aged 6 to 14 years, had psychiatric symptoms, 4.5 percent had conduct disorder followed by 3.25 percent children with mental retardation, 0.37 percent with depression, 1.87 percent psychotic symptoms and 2.87 percent with anxiety among the selected population.

Nair *et al.* (2004) conducted a community-based study on 899 school/ college students and school dropouts, aged 13 to 19 years, in Thiruvananthapuram, Kerala in India. For the assessment, BDI was used as a mood measuring instrument. It was found that 11.2 percent of school dropouts and 3 percent of school going young people had severe and extreme grades of depression.

Srinath et al. (2005) conducted a population-based study in urban, urban slum and rural areas of Bangalore, Karnataka in India whereby 2064 children, aged 0 to 16 years, formed the sample for the study. DISC-P, PIS and the FTN questionnaires were used for children, aged 6 to 16 years. Children between 12 to 16 years were also assessed using the DISC-C, Vineland Social Maturity Scale, Binet-Kamat Test, SLD battery and C-GAS. Prevalence rates of psychiatric morbidity among children, aged 0 to 16 and 4 to16 years, were 12.5 percent and 12.0 percent respectively. Among psychiatric morbidity, the prevalence of depression was 0.1 percent, conduct disorder was 0.2 percent, social anxiety and panic disorder was 0.1 percent each among 4 to16 years old population.

Ahmad et al. (2007) carried out a school based cross-sectional study in urban and rural areas of Aligarh, Uttar Pradesh in India, in which 410 male adolescents (205 from the rural schools and 205 from the urban schools), aged 10 to 19 years, were selected by PPS. The Y-PSC was used for screening of psycho-social impairment. Prevalence of overall psycho-social problems among the males, aged 10 to 19 years, was 17.9 percent (17.4% had educational difficulties, 9.2% had conduct disorders, 3.1% had depression and 3.8% had anxiety).

Various studies have been undertaken to assess the level of stress among adolescents whereas some studies have quantified the stress levels through mean stress score (assessed through different methods of measuring stress) (Latha & Reddy, 2007; Ghaderi, Kumar, & Kumar, 2009).

Dubat et al. (2007) conducted a study to assess the stress level among adolescent girls studying in 12th standard from Hisar and Hyderabad in India using Life Stress Scale. Findings of the study revealed that 47.5 and 72.5 percent of girls respectively were in the moderate category of family stress; financial stress was reported by 60 and 50 percent of girls respectively and

90 and 85 percent girls had moderate level of social stress among girls from two populations respectively.

A population-based study among 2048 adolescents, aged 12 to 16 years, from urban and rural areas of Goa in India was undertaken by Pillai et al. (2008). Mental disorders were diagnosed with the help of DAWBA tool. Findings of the study indicated that 1.8 percent adolescents, aged 12 to 16 years, had DSM IV disorders; 1.0 percent had anxiety disorders, 0.5 percent had depressive disorder, 0.4 percent had behavioural disorder and 0.2 percent had attention deficit hyperactivity disorder (ADHD).

An urban school based cross-sectional study was carried out by Bansal et al. (2009) on 125 students studying in 9th Standard in Pune, Maharashtra in India. The psychological instruments used for case detection were GHQ-12 and BDI. Results revealed that 18.4 percent of school going adolescents were depressed and 15.2 percent were distressed among the selected population.

Malhotra et al. (2009) undertook a six year follow-up prospective study on 727 adolescents, aged 10 to 17 years, from Chandigarh in India. Assessment done with the use of PIS and SDQ instruments revealed the incidence rate of psychiatric disorders to be 0.18 percent per year among the selected population.

Sahoo and Khess (2010) conducted a cross-sectional study in urban area of Ranchi city, Jharkhand, India. In this study, 500 young adult students were selected by stratified sampling method. DASS (Depression Anxiety Stress Scale) was used to assess the symptoms on dimensional basis and Mini International Neuropsychiatric Interview was carried out to diagnose the disorder on categorical basis. Depressive symptoms were present in 18.5 percent of the young adults, anxiety in 24.4 percent and stress in 20 percent of students. Clinical depression was present in 12.1 percent and generalized anxiety disorder in 19.0 percent of young population.

Deb et al. (2010) carried out a school-based study in urban area of Kolkata city, West Bengal in India in which 460 adolescents (220 boys and 240 girls), aged 13 to 17 years, was selected by multi-stage sampling technique. Self-reported semi-structured questionnaire and a standardized psychological test, the STAI, were used for assessment. It was found that 20.1 percent of boys and 17.9 percent of girls were suffering from high anxiety.

A study was undertaken by Sharma and Sidhu (2011) on adolescents, aged 16 to 19 years. A self-made questionnaire based on Bisht Battery of Stress was used to assess the prevalence of stress among this population. Findings revealed that 90.6 percent of population suffered from an academic stress.

According to World Health Report (2001), mental health disorders are one of the leading causes of disability worldwide. Three of the ten leading causes of disability in people between the ages of 15 to 44 years are mental disorders and the other causes are often associated with mental disorders.

In the light of above findings, WHO has recommended to promote mental health care services to address the psycho-social problems of adolescents through adolescent-friendly health care and counselling services which must be monitored on a continuous basis for its effective implementation (World Health Organization, 2013).

Alcohol Use

Use of alcohol among adolescents is another major concern in many countries. It reduces self-control and increases risky behaviors such as unsafe sex and dangerous driving. It is also a primary cause of injuries (including those due to road traffic accidents), violence (especially by a partner) and premature deaths. It can also lead to health problems in later life and affects the life expectancy. Setting a minimum age for buying and consuming alcohol and regulating how the alcoholic drinks are targeted at the younger market are among the strategies for reducing harmful drinking.

The United Nations Office on Drugs and Crime (UNODC) (2002) carried out a National Household Survey in rural and urban area of 24 States of India (excluding J&K) whereby 8,587 males, aged 12 to 18 years, were selected by systematic multi-stage stratified random sampling technique. Study specific questionnaire (drug dependence ICD-10) was developed and used for the collection of data for the survey. It was found that 21.4 percent male adolescents, aged 12 to 18 years, were alcohol users (UNODC, Regional Office for South Asia, 2002).

Other population based studies have shown that the prevalence of alcohol consumption varies from 1.3 to 15.6 percent across studies (Chaturvedi & Mahanta, 2004; Girish, Kavita, Gururaj, & Benegal, 2010; Ningombam, Hutin, & Murhekar, 2011; Medhi, Hazarika, & Mahanta, 2006) with a high consumption among males (12.6% to 20.7%) (Pagare, Meena, Singh, & Saha, 2004; Kangule, Darbastwar, & Kokiwar, 2011) and that too is more in urban (5.2%) as compared to rural (7.3%) areas (Tsering, Pal, & Dasgupta, 2010).

Pagare et al. (2004) carried out an observational study in urban area of Delhi in India among 115 male street children, aged 6 to 16 years. Semi-structured questionnaire was used for the study. Results of the observational study revealed that 12.6 percent male street children, aged 6 to 16 years, consumed alcohol.

Chaturvedi and Mahanta (2004) undertook a community based cross-sectional study in rural area of Changlang, Arunachal Pradesh in India. Simple random sampling method was used to select 1538 males and 1444 females in the age group 10 to 29 years. Study specific questionnaire was prepared and used for data collection. It was found that 11.2 percent of the individuals, aged 10 to 29 years, were alcohol users.

Medhi et al. (2006) conducted a population-based study in urban and rural areas of Dibrugarh, Assam in India among 2,264 individuals, aged 15 years and above, selected by multistage sampling design. Pre-designed and pre-tested questionnaire was used for the study. It was found that 32.2 percent of the individuals aged 15 years and above, consumed alcohol.

World Health Survey (2006) and International Institute for Population Sciences (IIPS) conducted a population-based survey in the states of Assam, Karnataka, Maharashtra, Rajasthan, Uttar Pradesh and West Bengal in India among 9994 individuals in 18-24 years' age group using a study specific questionnaire. It was found that 3.9 percent individuals, aged 18 to 24 years, were infrequent heavy drinkers and 0.6 percent was frequent heavy drinkers.

Rai et al. (2008) undertook a cross-sectional survey in urban area of Delhi, India among 3900 medical students, aged 17 to 32 years, using a study specific questionnaire. It was found that 32.1 and 9.7 percent of medical students, aged 17 to 32 years, had a lifetime and past month usage of alcohol respectively.

Parasuraman et al. (2009) carried out an All India National level study among 47,590 women and 24,997 men, aged 15-24 years. Structured questionnaire was prepared and used for the study. Results of the study revealed that 1 percent women and 11 percent men, aged 15 to 19 years and 1.4 percent women and 28.8 percent men, aged 20 to 24 years, consumed alcohol as per the findings of National Family Health Survey (NFHS-3).

A cross-sectional study was undertaken by Girish et al. (2010) in urban, rural and slum areas of Bangalore district, Karnataka in India. Simple random sampling method was used to select 28,507 subjects, aged 16 to 60 years, for the study. Data was collected using pre-tested semi structured questionnaire. Findings of this study revealed that 10 percent of alcohol users were adolescents and youth in the age group of 16 to 25 years.

Tsering et al. (2010) carried out a school based cross-sectional study in urban and rural areas of West Bengal, India in which 416 high school students studying in 8th, 9th and 10th standard was selected by multistage random sampling technique which constituted the sample population. Data was collected using pre-tested closed-ended self-administered questionnaire.

Results revealed that 5.2 percent urban adolescents and 7.3 percent rural adolescents were reported to be consuming alcohol.

A community based cross-sectional study was undertaken by Kangule et al. (2011) among 171 male youth, aged 15 to 24 years, selected by simple random sampling technique from the rural areas of Vasind, Andhra Pradesh in India. Pre-designed and semi-structured questionnaire was used for data collection. Results of the study revealed that 20.7 percent of males, aged 15 to 24 years, were using alcohol alone and 22.2 percent were using alcohol and tobacco together.

A school based cross-sectional survey carried out by Ningombam et al. (2011) among 1037 adolescents, aged 15 to 19 years, who constituted the sample population from urban areas of Imphal, Manipur in India. Self-administered questionnaire was used for data collection. It was found that 15.6 percent of adolescents, aged 15 to 19 years, had ever used alcohol.

A review at the national level was undertaken to study the harmful effects of alcohol consumption. Findings of the review indicated the greater social acceptability of drinking, its increasing consumption in rural and transitional areas, younger age of initiating drinking and phenomenal socio-economic and health impact more so among young people (Gururaj, Murthy, Rao, & Benegal, 2011).

Thus, the high risk behaviour which is linked to accidents, injuries and violence resulting into premature deaths as a consequence of harmful drinking among the young population is an increasing cause of concern in many countries (WHO, 2013).

Tobacco Use

The vast majority of people using tobacco today began consuming it when they were adolescents. Globally, at least 1 in 10 adolescents, aged 13 to 15 years, use tobacco although there are areas where this figure is much higher. WHO estimates of currently tobacco users to be more than 150 million adolescents and this figure is increasing globally at an alarming rate (World Health Organization, 2013).

National Family Health Survey (NFHS-3) revealed that 40 percent of males and 5 percent of females, aged 15 to 24 years, consumed tobacco nationwide. A median prevalence of tobacco use (ever users) was found to be 18.2 percent among 13 to 15 years old adolescents in India. The gender difference in the use of tobacco was significant. It was found to be 14 percent among males and 6.3 percent among females as estimated from a systematic review of 15 studies across India (Pal & Tsering, 2009).

Other studies have reported 9.8 to 20.3 percent life time prevalence of any tobacco products among adolescents (Singh, Pal, Mehta, & Kapil, 2007; Dhavan, Stigler, Perry, Arora, & Reddy, 2009). Gender differences for usage of any kind of tobacco ranged from 2.9 to 8.5 percent in boys and 1.5 to 9.8 percent in girls (Jindal, Aggarwal, Gupta, Kashyap, & Chaudhary, 2005). Gururaj and Girish (2007) have studied the prevalence of tobacco use among adolescents, aged 13-15 years, from Karnataka in India. Findings indicate the tobacco use to be 4.9 percent point prevalence and 5.1 percent life-time prevalence.

Global Youth Tobacco Surveys (GYTS) were carried out in the years 2006 and 2009 across India covering 13 to 15 years old adolescents in 180 schools. Findings of the surveys highlighted an increase in the current users of any form of tobacco from 13.7 to 14.6 percent and current users of cigarette from 3.8 to 4.4 percent from 2006 to 2009 (Gajalakshmi & Kanimozhi, 2010).

A school-based survey was undertaken in the urban area of Noida city, Uttar Pradesh in India. Sample comprised of 4786 students, aged 11 to 19 years. Self-administered questionnaire was used for data collection. Findings indicated 11.2 percent prevalence of any kind of tobacco use among 11 to 19 years old students, 8.8 percent prevalence of ever smokers (including current smokers), 4.6 percent prevalence of ever tobacco chewers (including current chewers), 3.7 percent prevalence of 'exclusive smokers' and 2.5 percent prevalence of 'exclusive tobacco chewers' (Narain, Sardana, Gupta, & Sehgal, 2011).

Data from several cited studies clearly point to the fact that though cigarette smoking seems to be decreasing among younger adolescents in some high-income countries, yet tobacco addiction is emerging as a big threat among young Indians. Prohibiting the sale of tobacco products to minors and increasing the price of tobacco products through higher taxes, banning tobacco advertisements and ensuring smoke-free environments are crucial to control the use of tobacco by adolescents.

Other Substance Use Disorders

Apart from tobacco and alcohol consumption, substance abuse is one of the major emerging problems among the young population that needs to be tackled effectively. The National Household Survey by UNODC showed that

3 percent of males consumed cannabis and 0.1 percent opiates (UNODC, Regional Office for South Asia; 2002), with common substances used being alcohol, tobacco, cannabis, cocaine and heroin (Chaturvedi, & Mahanta, 2004; Pagare, Meena, Singh, & Saha, 2004; Rai, Gaete, Girotra, Pal, & Araya, 2008; Sarangi, Acharya, & Panigrahi, 2008; Tsering, Pal, & Dasgupta, 2010; Bal, Mitra, Mallick, Chakraborti, & Sarkar, 2010; Ningombam, Hutin, & Murhekar, 2011; Kangule, Darbastwar, & Kokiwar, 2011).

Studies in India have also shown that non-tobacco substance abuse is common and nearly 30 percent among street children (Bal, Mitra, Mallick, Chakraborti, & Sarkar, 2010) with 57.4 percent of the male street children, aged 6 to 16 years, having indulged in it before coming to the observation home (Pagare, Meena, Singh, & Saha, 2004).

A school-based cross-sectional survey was carried out among 9319 students, aged 13 to 15 years, who were selected through two-stage cluster sampling method from Chandigarh and Punjab in India. Questionnaire with 85 items was prepared and used for the survey. The prevalence of ever-use of tobacco ranged between 2.9 to 8.5 percent among boys and 1.5 to 9.8 percent among girls in Chandigarh and Punjab respectively (Jindal, Aggarwal, Gupta, Kashyap, & Chaudhary, 2005).

Another study conducted by Sarangi et al. (2008) revealed the prevalence of substances abuse to be around 43 percent among young adolescents. In another study, it was reported to be 58.7 percent among students having used one or more substances at least once in life while 31.3 percent regularly use one or more substances (Juyal, Bansal, Kishore, Negi, Chandra., & Semwal, 2006).

Another school based cross-sectional study was undertaken by Reddy et al. (2006) among 11,642 sixth and eighth grade students from urban areas of Delhi and Chennai in India. Data was collected with the help of specifically designed questionnaire. Findings of the study showed that 24.8 and 6.7 percent of sixth-grade students and 9.3 and 2.9 percent of eighth-grade students had ever used tobacco and were current tobacco users respectively.

A cross-sectional survey among 4110 adolescents, aged 13-15 years from urban, transitional and rural areas of 12 districts of Karnataka, India was undertaken by Gururaj and Girish (2007). Three stage cluster sampling technique was used for selecting the sample. Study specific questionnaire was designed and used for collection of data. Point prevalence of tobacco use was 4.9 percent and lifetime prevalence was 5.1 percent among adolescents, aged 13 to 15 years.

Another cross-sectional study by Singh et al. (2007) was conducted on 3,422 children, aged 10 to 18 years from urban area of Delhi in India. Sample for the study was selected through population proportionate to size and simple random sampling methods. Pre-tested structured questionnaire was used for the study. It was found that 9.8 percent of adolescents had at least once experimented with any form of tobacco in their lifetime and 5.4 percent (boys: 4.6%, girls: 0.8%) of adolescents were "current users" of tobacco products.

A school based cross-sectional survey was undertaken by Mathur et al. (2008) among 11,642 students from 6th to 8th grade from urban area of Delhi and Chennai in India. A study specific questionnaire was used for the collection of data. Findings of the survey revealed that 18.9 percent for government school students and 12.2 percent for private school students have ever-used any of the tobacco products.

A systematic review of 15 studies in India involving 40062 students, aged 13 to 15 years, was carried out by Pal et al. (2009). Pre-tested A self-administered questionnaire was prepared, pre-tested and used for collecting the data. Findings revealed 18.2 percent median prevalence of ever users of tobacco among students, aged 13 to 15 years. Significant gender difference was found among the ever users of tobacco, the median prevalence being 14 percent among males and 6.3 percent among females.

An All India National Level study among 47,590 women and 24,997 men, aged 15 to 24 years, using structured questionnaire for data collection revealed that 40 percent of men and 5 percent of women, aged 15 to 24 years, and consumed tobacco nationwide while in Karnataka, 27 percent men consumed tobacco.

Another longitudinal school based study on a sample of 3404 students (1837 students in the 6th grade cohort and 1567 students in the 8th grade cohort) was carried out in urban area of Delhi and Chennai in India (Project MYTRI) which was followed up for 3 years. Self-administered questionnaire was used for surveys. Results of this study revealed that 10.5 percent of students in the year 2004, 15.4 percent in the year 2005 and 20.3 percent in the year 2006 reported lifetime use of any tobacco products (Dhavan, Stigler, Perry, Arora, & Reddy, 2009).

A school-based cross-sectional survey of nationally representative schools in India was undertaken by Gajalakshmi et al. (2010). Sample comprised of 11768 students, aged 13 to 15 years, selected in the year 2003 and 12,086 students were selected in the year 2006. Self-administered questionnaire was used for the surveys. Prevalence of current usage of any form of tobacco among 13 to 15 years old students reduced from14.6 to 13.7 percent; 4.4

percent of students currently smoked cigarettes in the year 2003 as compared to 3.8 percent in the year 2006.

Drug Use

Drug use among 15 to19 years' old adolescents is also an important global concern. The data from the National Health Survey in India suggested that about 0.1 percent of the male population in the age group of 12-60 years reported ever injecting any illicit drug. Injecting drug use was reported more often from the north east region of the country (UNODC, 2002).

Chaturvedi et al. (2004) reported that among 10 to 29 years old individuals, apart from tobacco and alcohol use, 2.2 percent of men and 0.3 percent of women were opium users in India. Data on prevalence of injecting drug users available in India showed that 5.6 and 14.4 percent of the males in the age group of 20 to 24 years and 25 to 29 years respectively were injecting drug users (Aceijas, Friedman, Cooper, Wiessing, Stimson, & Hickman, 2006). The use of prescription drugs (benzodiazepines and opiods) has also been a matter of great concern with its overuse being 16.2 percent (Rai, Gaete, Girotra, Pal, & Araya, 2008). Drug control may focus on reducing drug demand, drug supply or both and successful programs usually include structural, community and individual-level interventions.

Violence

Violence is also a leading cause of death in older adolescents, especially males. Interpersonal violence represents 43 percent of all adolescent male deaths in lower-income communities in the WHO Americas Region. Globally, 1 in 10 girls under the age of 20 years also report experiencing sexual violence.

Promoting and nurturing healthy relationships between parents and children early in life, providing training in life skills and reducing access to alcohol and fire arms can help to prevent injuries and deaths due to violence. Effective and empathetic care for adolescent survivors of violence and ongoing support can help deal with the physical and psychological consequences.

Injuries

Unintentional injuries are another leading cause of death and disability among adolescents. In the year 2015, over 1,15, 000 adolescents died as a result of road traffic accidents. Young drivers need advice on driving safely while laws that prohibit driving under the influence of alcohol and drugs need to be strictly enforced. Blood alcohol levels need to be set lower for teenage drivers. Graduated licenses for novice drivers with zero-tolerance for drunk-driving are recommended.

Drowning is also a major cause of death among adolescents. An estimated figure of 57, 000 adolescents, two-thirds of them being boys, is estimated to have drowned in the year 2015. Thus, teaching children and adolescents to swim is an essential intervention to prevent these deaths.

Suicide

According to the World Health Organization (WHO) estimates, about one million people commit suicide each year globally (WHO, 2013). In India, official reports indicate that nearly 1, 36, 000 persons voluntarily ended their lives in a suicidal act during the year 2011 (Ministry of Home Affairs, 2012). The official report also indicates that age specific suicide rate among 15 to 29 years old population is on the rise, its incidence rising from 3.73 to 3.96 per 1,00,000 populations per year during the period 2002 to 2011 (Ministry of Home Affairs, 2012).

Statistics indicate that about 40 percent of suicides in India are committed by individuals below the age of 30 years (Vijayakumar, 2006). The Million Death Study was undertaken by Patel et al. (2012) using RHIME (Representative, Re-sampled, Routine Household Interview of Mortality with Medical Evaluation) method. It was reported that the annual mortality rates among 15 to 29 years old was 25.5 and 24.9 per 1, 00,000 populations among males and females respectively.

Other studies have reported that the incidence of suicides among young population ranges from 100.1 to 72.2 per 1, 00,000 populations (Aaron, Joseph, Abraham, Muliyil, George, & Prasad, 2004). A study from Bangalore in India revealed that out of 5115 attempted suicides covering all age groups, 2.1 percent, 8.4 percent and 28.6 percent individuals were in the age group 10 to 15 years, 16 to 20 years and 21 to 25 years respectively; and of the 912 completed suicides, 2.2 percent, 16.2 percent and 21.6 percent were in the age group 10 to 15 years, 16 to 20 years and 21 to 25 years respectively (Gururaj, Sateesh, Rayan, Roy, & Amarnath, 2007).

Research findings reported by Aaron et al. (2004) indicate that 152 per 1,00,000 suicides have been reported among female adolescents in contrast to male adolescents among whom the incidence rate is 69 per 1,00,000. Similar findings have been revealed by other researchers (Patel, Ramasundarahettige, Vijayakumar, Thakur, Gajalakshmi, & Gururaj, 2012; Prasad, Abraham, Minz, Abraham, Joseph, & Muliyil, 2006). Soman et al. (2009) also indicated the incidence of suicide rates among males and females, aged 15 to 24 years, to be 5.1 and 8.1 per 1000 population per years respectively.

In India, the suicidal ideas and attempts were also reported to be high in Chandigarh (Arun & Chavan, 2009) and South Delhi (Sharma, Grover, & Chaturvedi, 2008) with nearly 6 percent of adolescents, aged 11 to 17 years and 15.8 percent of adolescents, aged 14 to 19 years, reporting suicidal ideas while 0.4 percent students, aged 11 to 17 years and 5.1 percent students, aged 14 to 19 years, reported suicidal attempts.

In United States, Bogg and Roberts (2004) conducted a meta-analysis of the leading behavioral contributors to mortality. To better understand the relationship of conscientiousness as a predictor of longevity, the authors conducted a meta-analysis of conscientiousness-related traits and the leading behavioral contributors (i.e. tobacco use, diet and activity patterns, excessive alcohol use, violence, risky sexual behavior, risky driving, suicide, and drug use) to mortality. This study demonstrated the importance of conscientiousness' contribution to the health process through its relationship to health-related behaviors.

Thus, mental health problems have emerged as an important but neglected issue of concern over the last decade. The probable reasons for adolescent morbidity and mortality could be that the focus towards psycho-social problems in Adolescent Health Programmes happens to be less as compared to Reproductive and Sexual Health Programmes in India. Thus, it is essential to give equal importance to other key areas like Mental Health Services and Behavioural Change Communication towards healthy lifestyle.

Strategies to Improve Mental Health Status of Adolescents

In view of the spectrum of mental disorders affecting the adolescents, the treatment depends upon their diagnosis and symptoms. As part of the treatment plan, the mental health professional/ psycho-therapist might decide a particular type of treatment or therapy either face to face or through the internet or may involve the family, teachers or peers as a part of treatment plan. The role of mental health professional or psycho-therapist is not to give advice but to enable the adolescent to make one's own decisions and find one's own solutions. Counselling is usually one to one therapy.

- **Psycho-Therapy:** It is based on talking to trained therapist. Also known as talk therapy, it helps the adolescents learn about their mental illness and help them deal with it effectively. It aims to get one to understand the problem. This is achieved by talking about one's thoughts and feelings and helping to change the way one thinks so as to enable one to manage one's problems in different ways. Psychotherapy is usually a one-to-one therapy but can also happen in groups (Corey, 2000).
- **Interpersonal Therapy:** Interpersonal Therapy (IPT) is a type of psycho-therapy based on the assumption that depression and interpersonal problems are inter-related. The goal of Interpersonal Therapy is to help an adolescent understand the social problems in relationships which lead one to get depressed or can put one at a risk of future depression.
- **Cognitive Behaviour Interventions:** The most frequently used individual and group treatment approaches, considered to be most effective, have a basis in Cognitive Behaviour Therapy (CBT). It is a structured psychological treatment that recognizes the way one thinks (cognition) and acts (behaviour) and affects the way one feels. CBT can be used to treat problems including anxiety, depression, low self-esteem, uncontrollable anger, substance abuse, eating disorders and other problems. The two most recognized theoretical Cognitive Behaviour approaches are Cognitive Behaviour Therapy (CBT) (Beck's1976;2000) and Ellis' Rational Emotive Behaviour Therapy (REBT) (Ellis,1977; Ellis & Harper,1975).

Although each of these approaches have distinctive features but both approaches require clients to identify their thoughts/ cognition that precede anger. The major in intervention common to both approaches is to help client determine whether these cognitions (thoughts)are rational or irrational, correct or false, distorted or accurate and to replace irrational, inaccurate thoughts with more rational and accurate ones.

- **Behaviour Therapy:** Behaviour Therapy is a major component of CBT. It is particularly useful for treatment of phobias or anxiety about being judged badly by others or an embarrassment in social situations.

The therapist helps to develop appropriate skills to deal with difficult situations and then use a step by step approach to help conquer the fears.

- **E-Therapies:** E-therapies are also known as online therapy or computer-aided psychological therapy. Therapies like Cognitive Behaviour Therapy and Behaviour Therapy also work well as e-therapies. Most e-therapies teach to identify and change the pattern of thinking and behaviour that might be stopping them from overcoming anxiety or stress. e-therapies work as good as face to face services for adolescents with mild to moderate depression and/or anxiety but not for adolescents in crises or for those who are seriously unwell.
- **Cognitive Behaviour Modification (CBM):** Is another major Cognitive Behaviour Therapy (CBT) that has been successfully used in treating anger. Like REBT and CBT, CBM shares the assumption that distressing emotions are typically due to maladaptive thoughts. CBM focusses on making client more aware of their self-talk and training them to develop self-talk that will enable them to cope more effectively in problematic situations (Meichenbaum's, 1977).
- **Stress Inoculation Training:** It is a particular coping skills program developed by Meichenbaum's (1985) to aid in stress reduction and has been demonstrated to be effective with a number of problems, including anger (Corey, 2000). SIT appears to be particularly beneficial when the client experiences anger in in relatively specific situations. in addition to help client learn behavioural techniques, he is taught a number of specific coping thoughts to assist in working through the anger provoking situations.
- **Assertive Training:** Before adolescents are taught behavioural assertiveness skills, they are frequently taught the difference between non-assertive, assertive and aggressive behaviour.in addition, any cognitive distortions or irrational thoughts impeding assertive behaviourr are replaced. Clients can learn assertive skills through modelling, role-playing and graded task assignments in real life situations (Lange & Jakubowski, 1976).
- **Self-Esteem Training:** Young adolescents with low self-esteem have lot of negative thoughts about themselves which are linked to negative emotions including sadness, anxiety, guilt and anger. This leads to mental health problems such as depression and also affects the social relationships. Effort should be made to boost the self-esteem of adolescents through online therapies or books.

- **Play Therapy:** Another valuable method for reducing anger problems is individual play therapy (Fischetti, 2001). Rather than accepting that one standardized play therapy approach is most effective for all clients and situations, Fischetti (2001) prefers a prescriptive approach that enables a counsellor to choose one they believe will be the most effective. Fischetti (2001) identifies three approaches i.e. Client-cantered play therapy which is non-directive approach; Release play therapy is a structured approach and Cognitive Behavioural Play Therapy (CBPT) which uses a wide range of behavioural techniques such as antecedents, reinforcers, contingencies, modelling, relaxation training, systematic desensitization and cognitive interventions etc. A frequent component of Cognitive behavioural play therapy is client homework.
- **Relaxation Training:** Anger may range from mild annoyance to violent rage which becomes a problem and needs treatment. Anger management can help them to get control over one's temper. Talking treatment such as CBT or counselling can work with anger management. Stress management and relaxation training can be a part of learning to manage anger. Adolescents can be taught to relax using a variety of modalities, including progressive relaxation, yoga, exercise or meditation.
- **Meditation:** Cheng (2016) reviewed 36 publications and suggested that integration of meditation is a potential, low cost, curative and non-intrusive method which can be inculcated in physical activities, music and art therapies and promotes adolescent's mental wellness.
- **Creative Therapies:** Art, music, dance or movement therapies are all forms of psycho-therapies that can help an adolescent cope with emotional, relationship or behavioural problems. Mental health professionals use these therapies to help adolescents communicate or express in new or more positive ways.
- **Classroom Based Educational Programs (CBEP):** These can be introduced in schools to improve mental well-being of students. Perry and Petrie (2014) studied the effect of classroom based educational resources on adolescent's mental health literacy and found that classroom based educational programme improved mental health literacy and reduced the stigma.
- **Family Therapies:** In case of adolescents undergoing mental illness, the family is often asked to participate in treatment as well. In such situations, families learn about the illness and its progression, methods

to support the adolescents through the recovery process and to avoid blaming and punishing them for behavior caused by mental illness. In such programmes, the family meets the therapist and the adolescent and discusses issues as a group. Besides, there are other things family members can do to help deal with adolescent mental illness.

- **Medication:** Some mental health problems can be treated with medication. Though it is not always a cure for problems but it can help control and improve symptoms. If a medical professional prescribes medication, it is usually combined with other therapies to help them to get better. Since different medications can have different side effects, staying fit and healthy can have an impact on mental health of adolescents.
- **Combination of Treatments:** Treatment usually involves psychotherapy, drug treatment and a combination of treatments directed at improving the home and school environment.

According to a study conducted by the National Institute of Health, 82 percent of depressed adolescents improved after combination of therapies/treatments and maintained their improved status for 36 weeks.

An article published in American Academy of Paediatrics suggests that parents of all adolescents must create a supportive, open atmosphere in which adolescents feel comfortable telling their parents whatever they intend and feel confident in sharing any information. Parents need to have open lines of communication with the adolescents so that they can assist if relapse occurs or the adolescents need some additional help.

WHO (2001) is strengthening the provision of mental health services through the implementation of mental health Gap Action Programme (mhGAP). The program aims at scaling up services for mental, neurological and substance use disorders for low and middle-income countries.

According to Comprehensive Mental Health Action Plan (CMHAP), (2013-2020), the four major objectives are to strengthen effective leadership and governance for mental health, provide comprehensive, integrated and responsive mental health and social care services in community-based settings, to implement strategies for promotion and prevention in mental health and to strengthen information services, evidence and research for mental health.

Therefore, this review helps to estimate the magnitude of psycho-social problem/dysfunction and its relationships with family-related factors along with various strategies to improve mental health status of adolescents residing in India and other developing countries. This aims to draw the attention of health planners and policy makers to focus on this significant but neglected aspect of adolescent health so as to plan and provide required adolescent health care services for optimum development of adolescents.

REFERENCES

Aaron, R., Joseph, A., Abraham, S., Muliyil, J., George, K., Prasad, J., ... Bose, A. (2004). Suicides in young people in rural southern India. *Lancet*, *363*(9415), 1117–1118. doi:10.1016/S0140-6736(04)15896-0 PMID:15064031

Aceijas, C., Friedman, S. R., Cooper, H. L., Wiessing, L., Stimson, G. V., & Hickman, M. (2006). Estimates of injecting drug users at the national and local level in developing and transitional countries, and local level in developing and transitional countries, and gender and age distribution. *Sexually Transmitted Infections*, *82*(Suppl. 3), iii10–iii17. doi:10.1136ti.2005.019471 PMID:16735287

Aggarwal, J. C. (2014). *Essentials of Educational Psychology*. Noida, India: Vikas Publishing House Pvt. Ltd.

Ahamd, A., Khalique, N., Khan, Z., & Amir, A. (2007). Prevalence of psychosocial problems among school going male adolescents. *Indian Journal of Community Medicine*, *32*(3), 219–221. doi:10.4103/0970-0218.36836

Ahmad, A., Khalique, N., Khan, Z., & Amir, A. (2007). Prevalence of Psychosocial problems among school going male adolescents. *Indian Journal of Community Medicine*, *32*(3), 219–221. doi:10.4103/0970-0218.36836

Anita, S., Gaur, D. R., Vohra, A. K., Subash, S., & Khurana, H. (2003). Prevalence of psychiatric morbidity among 6 to 14 years old children. *Indian Journal of Community Medicine*, *28*, 133–137.

Arumugam, B., Rajendran, S., & Nagalingam, S. (2013). Mental health problems among adolescents and its psychosocial correlates. *The Indian Journal of Medical Research*, *2*, 284–287.

Arun, P., & Chavan, B. S. (2009). Stress and suicidal ideas in adolescent students in Chandigarh. *Indian Journal of Medical Sciences*, *63*(7), 281–287. doi:10.4103/0019-5359.55112 PMID:19700908

Bal, B., Mitra, R., Mallick, A. H., Chakraborti, S., & Sarkar, K. (2010). Nontobacco substance use, sexual abuse, HIV, and sexually transmitted infection among street children in Kolkata, India. *Substance Use & Misuse, 45*(10), 1668–1682. doi:10.3109/10826081003674856 PMID:20590379

Bandura, A. (1977). *Social Learning Theory*. Prentice Hall.

Bansal, V., Goyal, S., & Srivastava, K. (2009). Study of prevalence of depression in adolescent students of a public school. *Industrial Psychiatry Journal, 18*(1), 43–46. doi:10.4103/0972-6748.57859 PMID:21234162

Beck, A. T. (1976). Cognitive Therapy and Emotional Disorders. International Universities Press.

Beck, A. T. (2000). *Prisoners of Hate: The Cognitive basis of Anger*. Perennial, NY: Hostility and Violence.

Bogg, T., & Roberts, B. W. (2004). Conscientiousness and Health-Related Behaviors: A Meta-Analysis of the Leading Behavioral Contributors to Mortality. *Psychological Bulletin, 130*(6), 887–919. doi:10.1037/0033-2909.130.6.887 PMID:15535742

Budhani, S. & Singh, B.B. (1996, July). Communication Support for Training Rural Youth in TRYSEM. *Indian Journal of Adult Education,* 33-37.

Cassey, R. (2010). The Storm and Stress of Adolescence: Insight from Human Imaging and Mouse Genetics. *Developmental Psychobiology, 52*(3), 225–235. PMID:20222060

Chaturvedi, H. K., & Mahanta, J. (2004). Socio cultural diversity and substance use pattern in Arunachal Pradesh, India. *Drug and Alcohol Dependence, 74*(1), 97–104. doi:10.1016/j.drugalcdep.2003.12.003 PMID:15072813

Cheng, F. K. (2016). Is Meditation Conducive to Mental Well-Being for Adolescents? An Integrative Review for Mental Health Nursing. *International Journal of Africa Nursing Sciences., 4*, 7–19. doi:10.1016/j.ijans.2016.01.001

Comprehensive Mental Health Action Plan (2013-2020). (n.d.). Retrieved from http://www.who.int/mental_health/action-plan_2013/en/

Corey, G. (2000). *Theory and Practice of Counseling and Psychotherapy* (6th ed.). Pacific Grove, CA: Brooks/Cole.

Crow and Crow. (1956). *Adolescent Development and Adjustment*. New York: McGraw –Hill Book Companies, Inc.

Deb, S., Chatterjee, P., & Walsh, K. M. (2010). Anxiety among high school students in India: Comparisons across gender, school type, social strata, and perceptions of quality time with parents. *Australian Journal of Educational and Developmental Psychology*, *10*, 18–31.

Dhavan, P., Stigler, M. H., Perry, C. L., Arora, M., & Reddy, K. S. (2009). Patterns of tobacco use and psychosocial risk factors among students in 6th through 10th grades in India: 2004-2006. *Asian Pacific Journal of Cancer Prevention*, *10*, 807–813. PMID:20104970

Dubat, K., Punia, S., & Goyal, R. (2007). A study of life stress and coping styles among adolescent girls. *Journal of Social Sciences*, *14*(2), 191–194. doi:10.1080/09718923.2007.11978373

Ellis, A. (1977). *Anger: How to Live with and Without it.* Citadel Press.

Ellis, A., & Harper, R. (1975). *A New Guide to Rational Living* (Rev. Ed.). Hollywood, CA: Wilshire Books.

Erikson, E. H. (1968). Reflections on the dissent of contemporary youth. *The International Journal of Psycho-Analysis*, *51*(1), 11–22. PMID:5533527

Fischetti, B. (2001). Use of Play Therapy for Anger management in the School Setting. In A. A. Drewes, C. e. Schaefer, & L. Caey (Eds.), *School-based play therapy* (pp. 238–255). New York: Wiley.

Gajalakshmi, V., & Kanimozhi, C. V. (2010). A survey of 24,000 students aged 13-15 years in India: Global Youth Tobacco Survey 2006 and 2009. *Tobacco Use Insights*, *3*, 23–31. doi:10.1177/1179173X1000300001

Ghaderi, A. R., Kumar, G. V., & Kumar, S. (2009). Depression, anxiety and stress among the Indian and Iranian students. *Journal of the Indian Academy of Applied Psychology*, *35*, 33–37.

Girish, N., Kavita, R., Gururaj, G., & Benegal, V. (2010). Alcohol Use and Implications for Public Health: Patterns of Use in Four Communities. *Indian Journal of Community Medicine*, *35*(2), 238–244. doi:10.4103/0970-0218.66875 PMID:20922099

Greenbaum, W. (1974). America in search of a new ideal: An essay on the rise of pluralism. *Harvard Educational Review*, *44*(3), 25–28. doi:10.17763/haer.44.3.68l73q37w4442j4q

Gururaj, G., & Girish, N. (2007). Tobacco use amongst children in Karnataka. *Indian Journal of Pediatrics, 74*(12), 1095–1098. doi:10.100712098-007-0204-x PMID:18174644

Gururaj, G., Murthy, P., Rao, G. N., & Benegal, V. (2011). *Alcohol related harm: Implications for public health and policy in India.* Publication No.: 73. Bangalore: National Institute of Mental Health & *Neurosciences*. Available from http://www.nimhans.kar.nic.in/deaddiction/CAM/Alcohol_report_NIMHANS.pdf

Gururaj, G., Sateesh, V. L., Rayan, A. B., Roy, A. C., & Amarnath, A. (2008). *Bengaluru injury surveillance collaborators group. Bengaluru injury / Road traffic injury surveillance programme: a feasibility study.* Bengaluru: National Institute of Mental Health & Neuro Sciences. Available from: http://www.nimhans. kar.nic.in/epidemiology/bisp/sr1.pdf

Hall, G. S. (1904). *Adolescence: Its Psychology and Its Relations to Physiology, Anthropology, Sociology, Sex, Crime, Religion, and Education: D.* New York: Appleton & Co.

Hall, G. S. (1904). Sources of Stress in High School College Preparatory and General Education Programs. Group Differences and Associations with Adjustment. *Adolescence, 44*(176), 925–948. PMID:20432608

Hurlock Elizabeth, B. (1976). *Child Development.* New York: The McGraw –Hill Companies, Inc.

Jellinek, M. S., Murphy, J., Little, M., Pagano, M. E., Comer, D. M., & Kelleher, K. J. (1999). Use of The Pediatric Symptom Checklist to Screen for Psychosocial Problems in Pediatric Primary Care: A National Feasibility Study. *Archives of Pediatrics & Adolescent Medicine, 153*(3), 254–260. doi:10.1001/archpedi.153.3.254 PMID:10086402

Jindal, S. K., Aggarwal, A. N., Gupta, D., Kashyap, S., & Chaudhary, D. (2005). Prevalence of tobacco use among school going youth in North Indian States. *The Indian Journal of Chest Diseases & Allied Sciences, 47*, 161–166. PMID:16022142

Juyal, R., Bansal, R., Kishore, S., Negi, K. S., Chandra, R., & Semwal, J. (2006). Substance use among intercollege students in district Dehradun. *Indian Journal of Community Medicine, 31*, 252–254.

Kangule, D., Darbastwar, M., & Kokiwar, P. (2011). A cross-sectional study of prevalence of substance use and its determinants among male tribal youths. *International Journal of Pharma and Bio Sciences*, *2*, 61–64.

Kessler, R. C., Berglund, P., Demler, O., Jin, R., Merikangas, K. R., & Walters, E. E. (2005). Lifetime prevalence and age-of-onset distributions of DSM-IV disorders in the national comorbidity survey replication. *Archives of General Psychiatry*, *62*(6), 593–602. doi:10.1001/archpsyc.62.6.593 PMID:15939837

Keyes, C. L. (2007). Promoting and protecting mental health as flourishing: A complementary strategy for improving national mental health. *The American Psychologist*, *62*(2), 95–108. doi:10.1037/0003-066X.62.2.95 PMID:17324035

Lange, A., & Jakubowski, P. (1976). *Responsible Assertive Behaviour: Cognitive/ behavioural proceduresfor Trainers*. Champaign, IL: Research Press.

Latha, K. S., & Reddy, H. (2007). Patterns of stress, coping styles and social supports among adolescents. *Journal of Indian Association for Child and Adolescent Mental Health*, *3*, 5–9.

Malhotra, S., Kohli, A., Kapoor, M., & Pradhan, B. (2009). Incidence of childhood psychiatric disorders in India. *Indian Journal of Psychiatry*, *51*(2), 101–107. doi:10.4103/0019-5545.49449 PMID:19823628

Malhotra, S., & Patra, B. (2014). Prevalence of child and adolescent psychiatric disorders in India: A systematic review and meta-analysis. *Child and Adolescent Psychiatry and Mental Health*, *8*(1), 22. doi:10.1186/1753-2000-8-22 PMID:25071865

Mathur, C., Stigler, M. H., Perry, C. L., Arora, M., & Reddy, K. S. (2008). Differences in prevalence of tobacco use among Indian urban youth: The role of socioeconomic status. *Nicotine & Tobacco Research*, *10*(1), 109–116. doi:10.1080/14622200701767779 PMID:18188751

Medhi, G. K., Hazarika, N. C., & Mahanta, J. (2006). Correlates of alcohol consumption and tobacco use among tea industry workers of Assam. *Substance Use & Misuse*, *41*(5), 691–706. doi:10.1080/10826080500411429 PMID:16603455

Meichenbaun, D. (1977). *Cognitive Behaviour Modification: An Integrative Approach*. New York: Plenum. doi:10.1007/978-1-4757-9739-8

Meichenbaun, D. (1985). *Stress Inoculation Training*. New York: Pergamon Press.

Michael, K. D., & Crowley, S. L. (2002). How effective are treatments for child and adolescent depression? Meta- analytic review. *Clinical Psychology Review*, *22*(2), 247–269. doi:10.1016/S0272-7358(01)00089-7 PMID:11806021

Ministry of Health and Family Welfare. (2014). *Launch of Rashtriya Kishor Swasthya Karyakram and National Consultation on Adolescent Health*. Available from: http://rksklaunch.in/rkskl-strategy.html

Ministry of Home Affairs. (2012). *Accidental deaths & suicides in India 2011*. New Delhi: National Crime Records Bureau. Available from: http://ncrb.nic.in/CD-ADSI2011/ADSI-2011%20REPORT.pdf

Muzammil, K., Kishore, S., & Semwal, J. (2009). Prevalence of psychosocial problems among adolescents in district Dehradun, Uttarakhand. *Indian Journal of Public Health*, *53*, 18–21. PMID:19806823

Nair, M. K., Paul, M. K., & John, R. (2004). Prevalence of depression among adolescents. *Indian Journal of Pediatrics*, *71*(6), 523–524. doi:10.1007/BF02724294 PMID:15226562

Narain, R., Sardana, S., Gupta, S., & Sehgal, A. (2011). Age at initiation & prevalence of tobacco use among school children in Noida, India: A cross-sectional questionnaire based survey. *The Indian Journal of Medical Research*, *133*, 300–307. PMID:21441684

National Family Health Survey (NFHS-3) 2005-06. (2007) *International Institute for Population Sciences (IIPS) and Macro International, India: Key Findings*. Mumbai: IIPS. Available from: http://www.measuredhs.com/pubs/pdf/SR128/SR128.pdf

NICE. (2008). *Promoting Children's Social and Emotional Well-Being in Primary Education*. Available from: https://www.nice.org.uk/guidance/ph12

NICE (2009). *Promoting Young People's Social and Emotional Well-Being in Secondary Education*. Academic Press.

NICE. (2010). *School-Based Interventions to Prevent the Uptake of Smoking Among Children and Young People*. Available from: http://www.nice.org.uk/nicemedia/pdf/PH23Guidance.pdf

Ningombam, S., Hutin, Y., & Murhekar, M. V. (2011). Prevalence and pattern of substance use among the higher secondary school students of Imphal, Manipur, India. *The National Medical Journal of India*, *24*, 11–15. PMID:21608351

Pagare, D., Meena, G. S., Singh, M. M., & Saha, R. (2004). Risk factors of substance use among street children from Delhi. *Indian Pediatrics*, *41*, 221–225. PMID:15064508

Pal, R., & Tsering, D. (2009). Tobacco use in Indian high-school students. *International Journal of Green Pharmacy*, *3*(4), 319–323. doi:10.4103/0973-8258.59740

Patel, V., Ramasundarahettige, C., Vijayakumar, L. J., Thakur, J., Gajalakshmi, V., Gururaj, G., ... Jha, P. (2012). Suicide mortality in India: A nationally representative survey. *Lancet*, *379*(9834), 2343–2351. doi:10.1016/S0140-6736(12)60606-0 PMID:22726517

Perry, Y., Petrie, K., Buckley, H., Cavanagh, L., Clarke, D., Winslade, M., ... Christensen, H. (2014). Effects of Classroom Based Educational Resource on Adolescents Mental Health Literacy: A Cluster Randomized Controlled Trial. *Journal of Adolescence*, *37*(7), 1143–1151. doi:10.1016/j.adolescence.2014.08.001 PMID:25151646

Pillai, A., Andrews, T., & Patel, V. (2009). Violence, psychological distress and the risk of suicidal behaviour in young people in India. *International Journal of Epidemiology*, *38*(2), 459–469. doi:10.1093/ije/dyn166 PMID:18725364

Pillai, A., Patel, V., Cardozo, P., Goodman, R., Weiss, H. A., & Andrew, G. (2008). Non-traditional lifestyles and prevalence of mental disorders in adolescents in Goa, India. *The British Journal of Psychiatry*, *192*(01), 45–51. doi:10.1192/bjp.bp.106.034223 PMID:18174509

Polaha, J., Dalton, T. W., & Allen, S. (2011). The prevalence of emotional and behavior problems in pediatric primary care serving rural children. *Journal of Pediatric Psychology*, *36*(6), 652–660. doi:10.1093/jpepsy/jsq116 PMID:21227909

Prasad, J., Abraham, V. J., Minz, S., Abraham, S., Joseph, A., Muliyil, J. P., ... Jacob, K. S. (2006). Rates and factors associated with suicide in Kaniyambadi block, Tamil Nadu, South India, 2000-2002. *The International Journal of Social Psychiatry*, *52*(1), 65–71. doi:10.1177/0020764006061253 PMID:16463596

Rai, D., Gaete, J., Girotra, S., Pal, H. R., & Araya, R. (2008). Substance use among medical students: Time to reignite the debate? *The National Medical Journal of India*, *21*, 75–78. PMID:18807312

Rani, M., & Karunanidhi, S. (2010). Prevalence of depressive symptoms among urban adolescents in South India. *Journal of Indian Association for Child and Adolescent Mental Health*, *6*(2), 33–43.

Reddy, K. S., Perry, C. L., Stigler, M. H., & Arora, M. (2006). Differences in tobacco use among young people in urban India by sex, socioeconomic status, age, and school grade: Assessment of baseline survey data. *Lancet*, *367*(9510), 589–594. doi:10.1016/S0140-6736(06)68225-1 PMID:16488802

Reddy, V. M., & Chandrashekar, C. R. (1998). Prevalence of mental and behavioural disorders in India: A meta-analysis. *Indian Journal of Psychiatry*, *40*, 149–157. PMID:21494462

Report, W. Y. (2003). *The Global Situation of Young People*. New York: Department of Economic and Social Affairs, United Nations. Available from: http://www.un.org/esa/socdev/unyin/documents/worldyouthreport.pdf

Sahoo, S., & Khess, C. R. (2010). Prevalence of depression, anxiety, and stress among young male adults in India: A dimensional and categorical diagnoses-based study. *The Journal of Nervous and Mental Disease*, *198*(12), 901–904. doi:10.1097/NMD.0b013e3181fe75dc PMID:21135643

Sarangi, L., Acharya, H. P., & Panigrahi, O. P. (2008). Substance abuse among adolescents in urban slums of Sambalpur. *Indian Journal of Community Medicine*, *33*(4), 265–267. doi:10.4103/0970-0218.43236 PMID:19876504

Sharma, J., & Sidhu, R. (2011). Sources of Stress Among Students Preparing In Coaching Institutes for Admission to Professional Courses. *The Journal of Psychology*, *2*(1), 21–24. doi:10.1080/09764224.2011.11885458

Sharma, R., Grover, V. L., & Chaturvedi, S. (2008). Suicidal behavior amongst adolescent students in south Delhi. *Indian Journal of Psychiatry*, *5*(1), 30–33. doi:10.4103/0019-5545.39756 PMID:19771304

Singh, S., & Gururaj, G. (2014). Health Behaviours & Problems Among Young People in India: Cause for Concern & Call for Action. *The Indian Journal of Medical Research*, *140*, 185–208. PMID:25297351

Singh, V., Pal, H. R., Mehta, M., & Kapil, U. (2007). Tobacco consumption and awareness of their health hazards amongst lower income group school children in National capital territory of Delhi. *Indian Pediatrics*, *44*, 293–295. PMID:17468526

Soman, C. R., Safraj, S., Kutty, V. R., Vijayakumar, K., & Ajayan, K. (2009). Suicide in South India: A community-based study in Kerala. *Indian Journal of Psychiatry*, *51*(4), 261–264. doi:10.4103/0019-5545.58290 PMID:20048450

Srinath, S., Girimaji, S. C., Gururaj, G., Seshadri, S., Subbakrishna, D. K., & Bhola, P. (2005). Epidemiological study of child & adolescent psychiatric disorders in urban & rural areas of bangalore, India. *The Indian Journal of Medical Research*, *122*, 67–79. PMID:16106093

Tsering, D., Pal, R., & Dasgupta, A. (2010). Licit and illicit substance use by adolescent students in eastern India: Prevalence and associated risk factors. *Journal of Neurosciences in Rural Practice*, *1*(2), 76–81. doi:10.4103/0976-3147.71721 PMID:21808508

UNODC, Regional Office for South Asia. (2002). *The extent, patterns and trends of drug abuse in India - National Survey*. Available from: http://www.unodc.org/pdf/india/publications/national_Survey/10_results.pdf

Valentine, C. W. (1957). Psychology and Its Bearing on Education, Vijayakumar, L. (2006). Suicide and mental disorders - a maze? *The Indian Journal of Medical Research*, *124*, 371–374.

Wittchen, H. U., Nelson, C. B., & Lachner, G. (1998). Prevalence of mental disorders and psycho-social impairments in adolescents and young adults. *Psychological Medicine*, *28*(1), 109–126. doi:10.1017/S0033291797005928 PMID:9483687

World Health Organization. (2001). *The World Health Report 2001. Mental Health: New Understanding, New Hope*. Geneva: WHO.

World Health Organization. (2011). *Young people: health risks and solutions. Fact sheet no. 345*. Available from: http://www.who.int/mediacentre/factsheets/fs345/en/index.html

World Health Organization. (2013). *10 facts on adolescent health*. Available from: http://www.who.int/features/factfiles/adolescent_health/facts/en/index4.html

World Health Organization. (2013). *Suicide prevention (SuPRE)*. Available from: http://www.who.int/mental_health/prevention/suicide/suicideprevent/en/

World Health Survey. (2006). *International Institute for Population Sciences (IIPS)*. World Health Organization (WHO). Available from: http://www.who.int/healthinfo/survey/whs_hspa_book.pdf

Chapter 4
Sexual and Reproductive Health

ABSTRACT

Around 1.2 billion people, or one out of every six persons of the world's population, are adolescents, aged 10 to 19 years. Most of them are presumed to be healthy, but there is still substantial premature death, illness, and injury among adolescents. Illnesses hinder the ability of adolescents to grow and develop to their full potential. Early pregnancy and child birth, unprotected sex, and/or exposure to HIV/AIDS and other sexually transmitted infections can jeopardize not only their current health but also their future health as adults and even the health of their future generations. Promoting healthy behaviors during adolescence and taking steps to better protect young people from health risks are critical for the prevention of health problems in adulthood and for the future health of coming generations as well as their ability to develop and thrive.

KEY FACTS

- Adolescents account for 23percent of the overall burden of disease (disability-adjusted life years) because of pregnancy and childbirth (Patton, Coffey, & Sawyer, 2009).
- An estimated 16 million births annually occur to young women aged 15-19 years, representing 11percent of all births (Sawyer, Afifi, & Bearinger, 2012).

DOI: 10.4018/978-1-5225-7384-5.ch004

- Almost all (95percent) of adolescent births take place in developing countries and 18percent and 50percent of births annually in Latin America and sub-Saharan Africa, respectively, occur during adolescence (Patton, Coffey, & Cappa, 2012).
- Approximately 2.5 million births occur to girls aged 12-15 years in low-resource countries each year of which around a million births occur to girls younger than 16 years in Africa (Neal, Matthews, & Frost, 2012).
- Globally, there are 44 births per 1000 adolescent girls, aged 15 to 19 years, per year (United Nations, 2012).

INTRODUCTION

Adolescence is often considered a period of relatively good health. However, adolescents (aged 10 to 19 years) face particular health risks, especially in relation to reproduction and sexuality. Eleven percent of all births and 14 percent of maternal deaths worldwide are among 15 to 19 years old females with 95 percent of adolescent births taking place in developing countries (Patton, Coffey, & Sawyer, 2009; WHO, 2011). Adolescents are also vulnerable to unwanted pregnancies; each year 7.4 million (International Planned Parenthood Federation; 2010) and 3 million girls experience unintended pregnancies and unsafe abortions respectively (WHO, 2011).

Adolescent pregnancy and its consequences represent a major public health concern in many low-middle income countries of the world. The World Health Organization has recently developed evidence-based guidelines addressing six areas: preventing early marriage; preventing early pregnancy through sexuality education, increasing educational opportunities and economic and social support programs; increasing the use of contraception; reducing coerced sex; preventing unsafe abortion; and increasing the use of prenatal care childbirth and postpartum care. In each of these areas, World Health Organization recommends directions for future research. This chapter provides an overview of global and regional initiatives that provide a window of opportunity for stepping up action in this important area (Chandra-Mouli, Camacho, & Michaud, 2013).

Early Pregnancy and Childbirth

Many adolescents become sexually active at an early age when they do not know how to avoid unwanted pregnancies and sexually transmitted infections. Contextual factors, such as the pressure to conform to media stereotypes and the norms of their peers, increase the likelihood of early and unprotected sexual activity.

First pregnancy at an early age is risky for the health of the mother as well as the newborn. Even though such births to adolescents account for 11 percent of all births worldwide, they account for 23 percent of the overall burden of DALY diseases (in terms of disability-adjusted life years) from pregnancy and childbirth among women of all ages (Patton, Coffey, & Sawyer, 2009).

The social consequences of pregnancy to adolescents include school dropout (with subsequent lower educational attainment and decreased social opportunities, including reduced lifetime earnings) and, in some settings, violence, including suicide and homicide (WHO, 2012).

In low- and middle-income countries (LMIC's), complications of pregnancy and childbirth are the leading cause of death in women, aged 15 to 19 years. The adverse effects of adolescent childbearing extend to the health of their infants. In low- and middle-income countries (LMIC's), stillbirths and deaths in the first week and first month of life are 50 percent higher among babies born to mothers younger than 20 years than those born to mothers aged 20 to 29 years. The younger the mother, greater is the risk (Patton, Coffey, & Sawyer, 2009).

The leading cause of death for 15 to 19 years' old adolescent girls globally is complications arising from pregnancy and childbirth. Nearly 11 percent of all births worldwide occur to adolescent girls, aged 15 to 19 years and the vast majority of these births are in low- and middle-income countries.

National Research Council and Institute of Medicine estimated 16 million births to mothers, aged 15 to 19 years, worldwide by the year 2008. About 95 percent of these births occurred in low- and middle-income countries (LMIC's) (National Research Council and Institute of Medicine, 2005). Births to younger adolescents were relatively less common, but according to recent estimates, 1 million births occur to girls, aged 12 to 15 years every year (Neal, Matthews, & Frost, 2012). Although adolescent birth rates are declining, the absolute number of births has declined lesser because of the increase in the size of the adolescent population (UNICEF, 2012).

The UN Population Division puts the global adolescent birth rate in the year 2015 at 44 births per 1000 adolescent girls. These age-wise variations in country rates range from 1 to over 200 births per 1000 adolescent girls, as per the Sustainable Development Goal (SDG) Indicators. However, these rates indicate a marked decline since the year 1990. This decline is reflected in a similar decline in maternal mortality rates among 15 to 19-year-old adolescent girls.

Adelson et al. (1992) reviewed the data available in New South Wales on teenage fertility rates and pregnancy outcomes. Teenage births comprise six percent of all births in New South Wales and these constitute a significant public health problem because these are associated with elevated rates of adverse pregnancy outcomes, which include low birth weight, perinatal death and pre-eclampsia. Risk is concentrated in females under 18 years of age. Pregnancy outcomes for females, aged 18 to 19 years, are similar to those of women, aged 20 to 24 years.

Scholl et al. (1994) reviewed the pregnancy complications and behavioral risk factors prevalent among teenage gravidas through meta-analysis of related studies. An increased risk of preterm delivery was associated with young maternal age in both developed and developing countries. Programs of comprehensive prenatal care appeared to have the potential to diminish risk of many complications. On the other hand, teenagers were at increased risk of maternal anemia, preterm birth and cesarean delivery in the developing world. Findings suggest that prenatal care regimens which provide social and behavioral services along with medical care could improve both the health of the mother and the offspring.

Coley et al. (1998) carried out a study with a focus on the dearth of knowledge concerning psychological precursors and consequences related to teenage pregnancy. Although the rate of teenage pregnancy has decreased substantially during this century, increasing rates of sexual activity, illegitimacy and welfare receipt raise public concerns. Findings suggest that many negative outcomes previously ascribed to mothers' age are as much related to teenage pregnancy as effects of it, although this claim is less substantiated regarding effects on children of teenage mothers.

In India, National Family Health Survey conducted a population-based study in rural and urban settings on 124,385 women, aged 15 to 49 years and 74,369 men, aged 15 to 54 years old populations during the years 2005-2006. Study specific questionnaire was developed and used. Results of the survey indicated that 4 percent of young women and 15 percent of young men had ever experienced sex before marriage and only 14.1 percent (14.7 percent urban versus 13.9 percent rural) of unmarried sexually active adolescent females used a contraceptive. Young people, aged 15 to 24 years, commonly engage in premarital sex more so in men (15-22 percent) as compared to women (1-6 percent) (National Family Health Survey, 2007; Kumar, Dandona, Kumar, & Dandona, 2011; anthya, Ram, Acharya, Mohanty, Jejeebhoy, & Singh, 2009; Alexander, Garda, Kanade, Jejeebhoy, & Ganatra, 2007; Savithri, Mehra, Kole, & Sakhuja, 2001).

Savithri et al. (2001) interviewed 354 girls and 467 boys, aged 15 to 19 years, and in an urban resettlement colony of Delhi in India in a community-based study. Results of the study indicated that 15 percent males and 6 percent females reported having premarital sex.

Alexander et al. (2007) conducted a community-based study in urban slum and rural settings of Pune, Maharashtra in India on 15 to 24 years old subjects using a study specific questionnaire. Results of the study showed that 16 to 18 percent of young men and 1 to 2 percent of young women had premarital sex.

Santhya et al. (2009) conducted a population-based survey in rural and urban settings of Andhra Pradesh, Bihar, Jharkhand, Maharashtra, Rajasthan and Tamil Nadu in India. A systematic, multi-stage sampling design was used to select 31,274 young women and 14,281 young men, aged 15 to 24 years, as the sample of the study. Survey was carried out with the help of study specific structured questionnaire developed for the purpose. Results of the survey revealed that 4 percent of young women and 15 percent of young men had ever experienced sex before marriage. Results also indicated that less than one percent of young men reported same-sex relations while relations with sex workers and married women were reported by one and three percent of young men respectively.

Sujay (2009) carried out a cross-sectional survey in three university settings in urban area of Gujarat, India whereby 3,202 college students, aged 15 to 24 years, were selected by stratified two stage random sampling technique. Self-administered questionnaires were used in the survey. Findings of the survey revealed that 39.7 percent males and 7.4 percent females reported having multiple-partner sex and 32.1 percent males and 3.2 percent females reported having paid/exchange (money/gift) sex.

A national level study was conducted in India by Gaffey et al. (2011) among 31040 men, aged 15 to 49 years, who were selected by multi-stage stratified cluster sampling technique used specifically prepared study specific questionnaire. Results revealed that among men, aged 15 to 24 years, 35.7 percent of unmarried, married or previously married men had sex with non-regular partners and 7.9 percent had sex with Female Sex Worker; 62.9 percent of unmarried men had sex with non-regular partners and 13.3 percent had sex with FSW; 6.5 percent of married men had sex with non-regular partners and 1.9 percent of married men had sex with FSW.

Ghule and Donta (2011) undertook an institutional based cross-sectional study in rural area of Thane, Maharashtra in India, in which 1500 students (800 males and 700 female), aged 5 to 24 years, were selected by random sampling method. Self-administered questionnaire was used for the study. Results of the study revealed that 11 percent boys and 1 percent girls reported penetrative sex (vaginal/oral/anal) and around half of them did not use condom. Homosexual experience was reported by 11 percent boys and 3 percent girls.

Kumar et al. (2011) carried out a population-based cross-sectional study in rural and urban areas of Guntur district, Andhra Pradesh in India which highlighted that 2,475 never married boys and girls, aged 15 to 24 years, were selected by systematic sampling technique. Interviews carried out on the sample population revealed that 21.7 percent males and 4.6 percent females reported that they had premarital sex. Out of this population, only 22.3 percent males and 6.3 percent females reported consistent condom use for premarital sex in the last six months.

Thus, high-risk sexual behaviour is a broad term covering early sexual activity, especially during adolescence and includes unprotected sex, except in a long-term, single-partner (monogamous) relationship, having multiple sex partners, having a high-risk partner (one who has multiple sex partners or other risk factors), exchange of sex (sex worker) for drugs or money, having anal sex or having a partner who does indulge in sex, except in a long-term, single-partner (monogamous) relationship and having sex with a partner who injects or has ever injected drugs. All these are known risk factors that put individuals at risk for contracting HIV/AIDS and a range of other sexually transmitted diseases like gonorrhoea, herpes, genital warts, Chlamydia, syphilis, trichomoniasis, etc.

HIV/AIDS

Adolescent girls are especially vulnerable to Human Immunodeficiency Virus (HIV) acquisition (Leclerc-Madlala, 2008). Poor, marginalized and disenfranchised youth suffer the highest burden of disease. For example, homeless adolescents face higher risks of HIV infection (Kissin, Zapata, & Yorick, 2007; Busza, Balakireva, & Teltschik, 2010). Adolescents with disabilities are particularly vulnerable to sexual abuse and resultant unplanned pregnancies and HIV and other sexually transmitted infections (STI's) (UNICEF, 2011).

Globally, more than 2 million adolescents are living with HIV/AIDS. Although the overall number of HIV-related deaths is around 30 percent since its peak in the year 2006, the estimates which suggests that HIV-related deaths among adolescents are rising over the years. This increase, which has been predominantly in the WHO African Region, may reflect the fact that although more children with HIV survive into adolescence, they do not all then get the care and support that they need to remain in good health and prevent transmission.

Trends in Sub-Saharan Africa (SSA) show that adolescent girls from the richest three quintiles have experienced declines in rates of pregnancy over time, whereas those from the poorest quintiles have faced increased rates (UNFPA, 2010).

An estimated 1,300,000 adolescent girls and 780,000 adolescent boys are living with Human Immunodeficiency Virus (HIV) worldwide (UNICEF, 2011). Over 800,000 young people are newly infected every year; 79 percent of these infections occur in Sub-Saharan Africa (SSA). Globally, young people account for 41percent of new infections among those, aged 15 years or older (UNAIDS, 2010).

Data from five countries in SSA with high rates of new HIV infections found that 7 to 31percent of boys and 9 to 58 percent of girls, aged 15-24 years, had been tested for HIV and received their results (UNICEF, 2011). Less than half of young men in Sub-Saharan Africa (SSA) reported using condoms at the time of the last sexual intercourse, and rates were even lower among young women (Millennium Development Goals Report, 2011).

In Sub-Saharan Africa, awareness with regard to their HIV status has been reported by only 10 percent of young men and 15 percent of young women, aged 15 to 24 years. Young people need to know how to protect themselves and must have the means to do so. This includes being able to obtain condoms to prevent sexual transmission of the virus and use of clean needles and syringes for those who inject drugs. In Sub-Saharan Africa (SSA), as many as 68 percent of adolescents have an unmet need for contraception (International Planned Parenthood Federation, 2010). Better accesses to HIV testing and counselling as well as stronger subsequent links to HIV treatment services for those who test HIV positive are also needed.

One of the specific targets of the health-related Sustainable Development Goal (SDG- 3) is that by the year 2030, there should be an end to the epidemics of HIV/AIDS, tuberculosis, malaria and neglected tropical diseases, hepatitis, water-borne diseases and other communicable diseases. Given the high prevalence of HIV/ AIDS in many countries, to achieve this Sustainable Development Goal, adolescents will need to be a central focus to control the epidemic of HIV/AIDS.

Sexual Violence

Gender-based violence is an all too common reality for many adolescents, especially girls. Globally, an estimated 30 percent of adolescent girls (15 to 19 years) experience intimate partner violence according to recent World Health Organization estimates (WHO, 2013).

Violence against women and girls increases the risk of adverse SRH outcomes including unintended pregnancy, acquisition of HIV and other sexually transmitted infections (STIs), as well as other adverse health outcomes such as the harmful use of alcohol and mental health disorders (e.g., depression) (United Nations Children's Fund; 2011; Garcia-Moreno, Jansen, & Ellsberg, 2006; WHO, 2010).

Female Genital Mutilation/Cutting (FGM/C) is a significant and widespread problem. According to recent estimates, about 125 million girls and women living in 27 African countries, Yemen and Iran have been subjected to this harmful traditional practice (United Nations Children's Fund; 2013). An estimated 3.3 million girls are at risk of undergoing FGM/C in Africa alone every year (Yoder, Wang, & Johansen, 2013).

Maternal Mortality and Morbidity

Early childbearing is linked with higher maternal mortality and morbidity rates (Blanc, Winfrey, & Ross, 2013; Nove, Matthews, & Neal, 2014; Ganchimeg, Ota, & Morisaki, 2014) and increased risk of induced, mostly illegal and unsafe, abortions (Shah, & Åhman, 2012). Maternal mortality and morbidity causes, thus, constitute the leading cause of death among adolescent females (WHO, 2011 a).

An analysis of data from 14 countries in Latin America for the period 1985 to 2003 found that adolescent girls, aged under 16 years, have four times higher risk of dying in pregnancy or childbirth than women aged 20 to 24 years (Conde-Agudelo, Belizán, & Lammers, 2005).

Adolescent pregnancy is independently associated with increased risks of low birth weight, preterm delivery, severe neonatal conditions, and early neonatal death (because of the increased risk of preterm birth) (Ganchimeg, Ota, & Morisaki, 2014). Of the estimated 22 million unsafe abortions that occur every year, 15 percent occur among young women aged 15 to19 years and 26 percent occur in those, aged 20 to 24 years (WHO, 2011b).

Furthermore, risky sexual behaviors and reproductive health problems in adolescence can have long lasting consequences into adulthood and into the subsequent generations. For example, impaired foetal growth is more common in pregnancies occurring before the age of 18 years and low birth weight is an important risk factor for adult-onset diabetes (Norris, Osmond, & Gigante, 2012).

Overall, improvements in adolescent health over the past five decades have not kept pace with those observed in children; mortality among 1 to 4-year-old children declined by more than 80 percent over the past five decades, whereas adolescent mortality rates only improved by 41 to 48 percent only (Viner, Coffey, & Mathers, 2011).

The International Conference on Population and Development (ICPD) Program of Action (PoA) describes services included under the umbrella of Sexual And Reproductive Health Services (SRHS), such as family-planning counselling and services; prenatal and postnatal care and delivery; abortion services and post-abortion care; treatment and prevention of reproductive tract and sexually transmitted diseases and infections including HIV and information and counselling about human sexuality (United Nations, 1995).

Rights of Adolescents

The rights of children (people under 18 years of age) to survive, grow and develop are enshrined in International legal documents. In the year 2013, the Committee on the Rights of the Child (CRC) which oversees the child rights convention, published guidelines on the right of children and adolescents to the enjoyment of the highest attainable standards of health and a general comment on realizing the rights of children during adolescence was published in the year 2016. It highlights the obligations to recognize the special health and developmental needs and rights of adolescents and young people. The Convention on the Elimination of Discrimination against Women (CEDAW) also sets out the rights of women and girls to health and adequate health care.

The concepts of Sexual and Reproductive Health (SRH) and of reproductive rights were adopted for the first time by governments under the aegis of the United Nations at the International Conference on Population and Development (ICPD) in Cairo in 1994. International Conference on Population and Development (ICPD) laid out a bold, clear, and comprehensive definition of reproductive health as,

...a state of complete physical, mental and social wellbeing and not merely the absence of disease or infirmity, in all matters relating to the reproductive system and to its functions and processes. (United Nations, 1995)

The ICPD Programme of Action (PoA) was forward looking in many areas of SRH and rights and notably in relation to adolescents and young people. It called for "meeting the educational and service needs of adolescents to enable them to deal in a positive and responsible way with their sexuality." It also stressed that reproductive health services should be made accessible through primary health care systems to individuals of all appropriate ages, including adolescents, as soon as possible and no later than the year 2015 (United Nations, 1995).

At the ICPD and its 5-year review in 1999, governments recognized that investing in the health of adolescents is important not only for the well-being of adolescents but also for the current and future well-being of the communities and societies. Confirming the critical importance of Adolescent Sexual and Reproductive Health and Rights (ASRHR), the Commission on Population and Development in the year 2012 issued some of the strongest language on the reproductive rights of young people to emerge from a global intergovernmental negotiation.

Key points of the final resolution included the right of young people to Comprehensive Sexuality Education (CSE), to decide on all matters related to their sexuality; access to SRH services, including safe abortion where legal, that respect confidentiality and do not discriminate; and the protection and promotion of young people's right to control their sexuality free from violence, discrimination, and coercion (United Nations, 2012).

In the year 2014, the International Health and Development Community (IHDC) reviewed the 20 years of progress made in implementing the ICPD Programme of Action (PoA), and further in the year 2015, a new set of sustainable development goals were established for a post-2015 development agenda. New global agendas were set, which will shape funding decisions and country programs for several years. There are calls by some stakeholders for stand-alone goals on adolescents and youth in the post-2015 agenda, whereas the General Assembly's Open Working Group (GAOWG) on Sustainable Development Goals (SDG), among others, has indicated that youth concerns need to be reflected across goals. There are also strong calls for adolescents and young people to take an active part in shaping and monitoring this agenda.

One of the specific targets of the Sustainable Development Goal (SDG-3) in relation to health of adolescents is that by the year 2030, the world should ensure universal access to sexual and reproductive health-care services, including for family planning, information and education, and the integration of reproductive health of adolescents into national strategies and programs.

To support this, a proposed indicator for the Global Strategy for Women's, Children's and Adolescents' Health (GSWCAH) is the adolescent birth rate. Better access to contraceptive information and services can reduce the number of adolescent girls becoming pregnant and giving birth at too young an age. Laws that specify a minimum age of marriage at 18 years and which are enforced can help reduce the risk of teenage pregnancies. Adolescent girls, who become pregnant, need an access to quality antenatal care. Where permitted by law, adolescents who opt to terminate their pregnancies should have an access to safe abortion.

WHO Response

In May 2017, WHO published a major report: *Global Accelerated Action for the Health of Adolescents (GAA-HA): Guidance to support country implementation.* The GAA-HA Guidance has drawn on inputs received during extensive consultations with its member states, United Nations agencies, adolescents and young people, civil society and other partners. It aims to assist governments in deciding what they plan to do and how they plan to do it as they respond to the health needs of adolescents in their countries. This reference document targets national level policymakers and program managers to assist them in planning, implementing, monitoring and evaluation of adolescent health programs.

Overall, WHO carries out a wide range of functions to improve the health of young people including production of evidence-based guidelines to support health services and other sectors; making recommendations to governments on adolescent health and the provision of high quality age-appropriate health services for adolescents; documenting progress in adolescent health and development and raising awareness on health issues for young people among the general public and other interested stakeholders.

Efforts in recent years have focused on not only ensuring health service availability but also making its provision adolescent friendly that is, accessible, acceptable, equitable, appropriate, and effective (WHO, 2009). These efforts aim to increase the ability and willingness to obtain services, particularly among those adolescents who need them the most.

There is considerable variability among LMIC's on whether premarital sexuality can be discussed in a meaningful way. This presents a major challenge for programs. Stakeholders need to be engaged to develop culturally acceptable mechanisms to reduce pregnancy and the associated negative health outcomes.

Curriculum-based sexuality education should be implemented. These programs will be more effective if they develop life skills, address contextual factors, and focus on the emerging feelings and experiences that accompany sexual and reproductive maturity. Sexuality education programs should be encouraged to link with reproductive health services, notably contraceptive services.

Future research in this area should focus on building evidence on the effect of interventions that increase employment, school retention, education availability and social supports. Research should be conducted across socio-cultural contexts to identify feasible, scalable interventions to reduce early pregnancy among adolescents.

REFERENCES

Adelson, P. L., Frommer, M. S., Pym, M. A., & Rubin, G. L. (1992). Teenage pregnancy and fertility in New South Wales: An examination of fertility trends, abortion and birth outcomes. *Australian Journal of Public Health, 16*(3), 238–244. doi:10.1111/j.1753-6405.1992.tb00061.x PMID:1482715

Adolescent Health. (n.d.). Retrieved from http://www.who.int/mediacentre/factsheets/fs345/en/

Alexander, M., Garda, L., Kanade, S., Jejeebhoy, S., & Ganatra, B. (2007). Correlates of premarital relationships among unmarried youth in Pune district, Maharashtra, India. *International Family Planning Perspectives, 33*(04), 150–159. doi:10.1363/3315007 PMID:18178539

Blanc, A. K., Winfrey, W., & Ross, J. (2013). New Findings for maternal mortality age patterns: Aggregated results for 38 countries. *PLoS One, 8*(4), e59864. doi:10.1371/journal.pone.0059864 PMID:23613716

Busza, J. R., Balakireva, O. M., Teltschik, A., Bondar, T. V., Sereda, Y. V., Meynell, C., & Sakovych, O. (2010). Street-based adolescents at high risk of HIV in Ukraine. *Journal of Epidemiology and Community Health, 65*(12), 1166–1170. doi:10.1136/jech.2009.097469 PMID:20864455

Chandra-Mouli, V., Camacho, A. V., & Michaud, P. A. (2013). WHO guidelines on preventing early pregnancy and poor reproductive outcomes among adolescents in developing countries. *The Journal of Adolescent Health, 52*(5), 517–522. doi:10.1016/j.jadohealth.2013.03.002 PMID:23608717

Coley, L., & Chase-Lansdale, P. L. (1998). Adolescent pregnancy and parenthood: Recent evidence and future directions. *The American Psychologist, 53*(2), 152–166. doi:10.1037/0003-066X.53.2.152 PMID:9491745

Conde-Agudelo, A., Belizán, J. M., & Lammers, C. (2005). Maternal-perinatal morbidity and mortality associated with adolescent pregnancy in Latin America: A Cross-sectional study. *American Journal of Obstetrics and Gynecology, 192*(2), 342–349. doi:10.1016/j.ajog.2004.10.593 PMID:15695970

Gaffey, M.F., Venkatesh, S., Dhingra, N., Khera, A., Kumar, R., & Arora, P. (2011). Male use of female sex work in India: A Nationally Representative behavioural Survey. *Plos One, 6,* e 22704.

Ganchimeg, T., Ota, E., Morisaki, N., Laopaiboon, M., Lumbiganon, P., Zhang, J., ... Mori, R. (2014). Pregnancy and childbirth outcomes among adolescent mothers: A World Health Organization multi-country study. *British Journal of Obstetrics and Gynaecology, 121*(Supplement s1), 40–48. doi:10.1111/1471-0528.12630 PMID:24641534

Garcia-Moreno, C., Jansen, H. A., Ellsberg, M., Heise, L., & Watts, C. H. (2006). Prevalence of intimate partner violence: Findings from the WHO multi-country study on women's health and domestic violence. *Lancet, 368*(9543), 1260–1269. doi:10.1016/S0140-6736(06)69523-8 PMID:17027732

Ghule, M., & Donta, B. (2011). Correlates of sexual behaviour of rural college youth in Maharashtra, India. *Eastern Journal of Medicine, 16*, 122–132.

International Planned Parenthood Federation. (2010). *Facts on the sexual and reproductive health of adolescent women in the developing world.* Guttmacher Institute.

Kissin, D. M., Zapata, L., Yorick, R., Vinogradova, E. N., Volkova, G. V., Cherkassova, E., ... Hillis, S. (2007). HIV seroprevalence in street youth, St. Petersburg, Russia. *AIDS (London, England)*, *21*(17), 2333–2340. doi:10.1097/QAD.0b013e3282f125b3 PMID:18090282

Kumar, G. A., Dandona, R., Kumar, S. G., & Dandona, L. (2011). Behavioral surveillance of premarital sex among never married young adults in a high HIV prevalence district in India. *AIDS and Behavior*, *15*(1), 228–235. doi:10.100710461-010-9757-1 PMID:20625924

Leclerc-Madlala, S. (2008). Age-disparate and intergenerational sex in southern Africa: The dynamics of hyper-vulnerability. *AIDS (London, England)*, *22*(4), S17–S25. doi:10.1097/01.aids.0000341774.86500.53 PMID:19033752

Millennium Development Goals Report. (2011). United Nations.

National Family Health Survey (NFHS-3) (2005-06). (2007). *International Institute for Population Sciences (IIPS) and Macro International: Key Findings*. Mumbai: IIPS. Available from: http://www.measuredhs.com/pubs/pdf/SR128/SR128.pdf

National Research Council and Institute of Medicine. (2005). *Growing up global: The changing transitions to adulthood in developing countries*. Washington, DC: The National Research Council and Institute of Medicine.

Neal, S., Matthews, Z. E., Frost, M., Fogstad, H., Camacho, A., & Laski, L. (2012). Child bearing in adolescents aged 12-15 years in low resource countries: A neglected issue. New estimates form demographic and household surveys in 42 countries. *Acta Obstetricia et Gynecologica Scandinavica*, *91*(9), 1114–1118. doi:10.1111/j.1600-0412.2012.01467.x PMID:22620274

Norris, S. A., Osmond, C., Gigante, D., Kuzawa, C. W., Ramakrishnan, L., Lee, N. R., ... Fall, C. H. D. (2012). Size at birth, weight gain in infancy and childhood, and adult diabetes risk in five low- or middle-income country birth cohorts. *Diabetes Care*, *35*(1), 72–79. doi:10.2337/dc11-0456 PMID:22100968

Nove, A., Matthews, Z., Neal, S., & Camacho, A. V. (2014). Maternal mortality in adolescents compared with women of other ages: Evidence from 144 countries. *The Lancet. Global Health*, *2*(3), e155–e164. doi:10.1016/S2214-109X(13)70179-7 PMID:25102848

Patton, G. C., Coffey, C., Cappa, C., Currie, D., Riley, L., Gore, F., ... Ferguson, J. (2012). Health of the world's adolescents: A synthesis of internationally comparable data. *Lancet*, *379*(9826), 1665–1675. doi:10.1016/S0140-6736(12)60203-7 PMID:22538181

Patton, G. C., Coffey, C., Sawyer, S. M., Viner, R. M., Haller, D. M., Bose, K., ... Mathers, C. D. (2009). Global patterns of mortality in young People: A systematic analysis of population data. *Lancet*, *374*(9693), 881–892. doi:10.1016/S0140-6736(09)60741-8 PMID:19748397

Santhya, K. G., Ram, U., Acharya, R., Mohanty, S., Jejeebhoy, S. J., & Singh, A. (2009). Pre-marital sexual relations among youth in India: findings from the youth in India, situations and needs study. *Proceedings of the xxvI International Union for the Scientific Study of Population Conference.*

Savithri, R., Mehra, S., Kole, S. K., & Sakhuja, A. (2001). *Sexual behaviour among adolescents and young people in India: some emerging trends*. Working Paper Series No. 3. New Delhi: MAMTA -Health Institute for Mother and Child.

Sawyer, S. M., Afifi, R. A., Bearinger, L. H., Blakemore, S.-J., Dick, B., Ezeh, A. C., & Patton, G. C. (2012). Adolescence: A foundation for future health. *Lancet*, *379*(9826), 1630–1640. doi:10.1016/S0140-6736(12)60072-5 PMID:22538178

Scholl, T. O., Hediger, M. L., & Belsky, D. H. (1994). Prenatal care and maternal health during adolescent pregnancy: A review and meta-analysis. *The Journal of Adolescent Health*, *15*(6), 444–456. doi:10.1016/1054-139X(94)90491-K PMID:7811676

Shah, I. H., & Åhman, E. (2012). Unsafe abortion differentials in 2008 by age and developing country region: High burden among young women. *Reproductive Health Matters*, *20*(39), 169–173. doi:10.1016/S0968-8080(12)39598-0 PMID:22789095

Sujay, R. (2009). *Premarital sexual behaviour among unmarried college students of Gujarat, India*. Health and Population Innovation, Fellowship Programme Working Paper No. 9.

Sustainable Development Goal Indicators. (n.d.). *Global Database*. Retrieved from https://unstats.un.org/sdgs/indicators/database/?indicator=3.7.2

UNAIDS. (2010). *Global report: UNAIDS report on the global AIDS epidemic*. Geneva: Joint United Nations Programme on HIV/AIDS.

UNFPA. (2010). *How universal is access to reproductive health? A review of the evidence*. New York: United Nations Population Fund.

UNICEF. (2011). *Opportunity in crisis: Preventing HIV from early adolescence to early adulthood*. New York: United Nations Children's Fund.

UNICEF. (2012). *Progress for children. A report card for adolescents*. New York: UNICEF.

United Nations. (1995). *Population and development: Programme of action adopted at the International Conference on Population and Development, Dept. for Economic and Social Information and Policy Analysis*. New York: UN.

United Nations. (2012). *Commission on population and development resolution 2012/1 adolescents and youth, report on the forty fifth session*. UN Doc E/2012/25, E/CN.9/2012/8.

United Nations Children's Fund. (2011). *Opportunity in crisis: Preventing HIV from early adolescence to early adulthood*. New York: United Nations Children's Fund.

United Nations Children's Fund. (2013). *Female genital mutilation/cutting: A statistical overview and exploration of the dynamics of change*. New York: United Nations Children's Fund.

Viner, R. M., Coffey, C., Mathers, C., Bloem, P., Costello, A., Santelli, J., & Patton, G. C. (2011). 50-Year mortality trends in children and young people: A study of 50 low-income, middle-income, and high income countries. *Lancet*, *377*(9772), 1162–1174. doi:10.1016/S0140-6736(11)60106-2 PMID:21450338

World Health Organization. (2009). *Quality assessment guidebook: A guide to assessing health services for adolescent clients*. Geneva: WHO.

World Health Organization. (2010). *Preventing intimate partner and sexual violence against women: Taking action and generating evidence*. Geneva: World Health Organization.

World Health Organization. (2011). *Mortality estimates by cause, age, and sex for the year*. Geneva: WHO.

World Health Organization. (2011). *Preventing early pregnancy: What the evidence says?* Geneva: WHO.

World Health Organization. (2011a). *Preventing early pregnancy and poor reproductive outcomes among adolescents in developing countries.* World Health Organization.

World Health Organization. (2011b). *Mortality estimates by cause, age, and sex for the year 2008.* Geneva: World Health Organization.

World Health Organization. (2012). Early marriages, adolescent and young pregnancies. Report by the Secretariat. A 65/13. Geneva, Switzerland: WHO.

World Health Organization. (2013). *Global and regional estimates of violence against women: Prevalence and health effects of intimate partner violence and non-partner sexual violence.* Geneva: World Health Organization.

World Health Organization. (2013). *10 facts on adolescent health.* Available from: http://www.who.int/features/factfiles/adolescent_health/facts/en/index4.html

World Health Organization. (2013). *Suicide prevention (SuPRE).* Available from: http://www.who.int/mental_health/prevention/suicide/suicideprevent/en/

Yoder, P. S., Wang, S., & Johansen, E. (2013). Estimates of female genital mutilation/cutting in 27 African countries and Yemen. *Studies in Family Planning*, *44*(2), 189–204. doi:10.1111/j.1728-4465.2013.00352.x PMID:23720002

Chapter 5 Adolescent Health Management

ABSTRACT

The present state of affairs of adolescent health status clearly shows that the condition of today's youth has significantly deteriorated as revealed by severe malnutrition, poor reproductive health, high aggression, increased depression, increased suicidal rates, drug use, substance abuse, etc., which are the clear indications of the challenges that adolescents are facing. No doubt that they are at risk because they lack social support to seek accurate information and services. In such a scenario, there is an urgent need to provide today's youth with new set of ways and systems to deal with the changing demands of life. It is essential that the adolescents be helped to develop skills inherently to handle a wide variety of choices, changes, and the stressors. It calls for a need of life skill education for adolescents so as to enable them to develop psycho-social competencies and interpersonal skills which help them to make informed decisions, communicate effectively, and develop coping and self-management skills so as to enable them to lead a healthy and productive life.

KEY FACTS

- Recent studies show that there is a significant rise in the problems faced by the adolescents for example, serious emotional disturbances have increased (WHO, 2001).

DOI: 10.4018/978-1-5225-7384-5.ch005

- Increased sexual activity among school going adolescents, rise in HIV/ AIDS cases in India as well as greater use of alcohol consumption has been found (BSS, 2007).
- Apart from the above, use of heavy drugs and youth drop outs has also increased in the recent years (UNICEF, 2001).

INTRODUCTION

Adolescence is a transitional period of development between childhood and adulthood which is accompanied by physical, sexual, psychological and social changes. Adolescence is often described as an exciting transitory phase in the human life cycle but is perhaps the most challenging phase as well. This is a time when adolescents evolve into adults with newly discovered independence and renewed responsibilities. They are constantly in search of their own new identity. They tend to question and appreciate the values of the adult life and try to assert their identity. During adolescence, they develop various skills that help them to grow into caring and responsible adults. When adolescents are supported and encouraged by caring adults, they thrive in unimaginable ways, becoming resourceful and contributing members of their families and societies. Adolescents are, thus, considered as the productive members of a society.

During the 21st century, life itself is undergoing significant transition and also the tremendous changes in all spheres occurring throughout the world. Among the most affected ones are the adolescents. Today, greater complexities of lifestyle, uncertainty and diversity, more and more peer as well as societal pressures, rapid changes in the home and the school environment as well as the continued deprivation put adolescents at the crossroads of their lives, thus facing an uncertain future in undertaking the responsibilities of adulthood and to enter the world of work. Now-a-days, the lives of adolescents are becoming miserable due to many reasons, including an inappropriate home and school environment. They are becoming individuals who are less motivated, less confident and less secure and are thus engaging in anti-social activities and spoiling their valuable lives.

Rapidly changing personal, social, moral, ethical and religious values have ushered certain 'life styles changes' in the present society, especially among the adolescents. Certain inbuilt buffers of the society, which used to serve as both support and control, are no longer available to the adolescents of present times, for instance the extended family system, the smaller community that had personal and closed uniform culture in the smaller circle of living, traditional ways of thinking and practicing etc. The stress faced by the adolescents in such a current situation is enormous. This is reflected by growing crime and rising suicide rates among young adolescents.

The present knowledge of adolescent's health status clearly shows that the condition of today's youth has significantly deteriorated. Recent studies show that there is a significant rise in the problems faced by the adolescents for example, serious emotional disturbances have increased (WHO, 2001), increased sexual activity among school going adolescents, rise in HIV/AIDS cases in India as well as greater use of alcohol consumption has been found (BSS, 2007). Apart from the above, use of heavy drugs and youth drop outs has also increased in the recent years (UNICEF, 2001).

All these studies clearly illustrate the increase in aggressiveness, depression, suicidal cases, drug use and depressive symptoms among adolescents. Information overload, mixed messages from media, press, teachers and the family as well as from the society at large add to the confusing scenario of the assimilating young minds. No doubt that they are at risk because they lack social support to seek accurate information and services. This gives the clear image of the struggle that the adolescents go through as well as the problems and challenges faced by them. Thus, providing an experience that would strengthen adolescent's coping abilities to counter environmental stress and disadvantages with which they sometimes have to cope with while experiencing is the need of the hour.

Nair (2005) in his article wrote that adolescence is a period of experiencing and expanding. Adolescents need help and guidance in decision making, problem solving, critical thinking, developing interpersonal skills, self-awareness and empathy in coping with the stress and managing their emotions. Beneath frequent violent outbursts, sudden mood swings and related interpersonal problems of an adolescent, there may be a person crying out for a professional help. Extra care is needed while offering help to adolescents' problems because it is not easy for them to accept the fact that they need professional help.

In such a scenario, there is an urgent need to provide today's youth with new set of ways and systems to deal with the changing demands of life. Since the 'individual' rather than the 'system' is recognized as the basic unit of the society, it is essential that the adolescents be helped to develop skills inherently to handle a wide variety of choices, changes and the stressors.

One best practice model for contributing to the healthy development of adolescents is a life skills approach. A key aspect of human development - as important to basic survival as intellect - is the acquisition of socio-cognitive and emotional coping skills. This has been shown to have an impact on behavior of adolescents.

For more than a decade, researches on interventions that address these specific socio-cognitive and emotional coping skill areas have shown the effectiveness of these skills in promoting desirable behaviors such as sociability, improved communication, effective decision making and conflict resolution as well as preventing negative or high-risk behaviors such as use of tobacco, alcohol and other drugs, unsafe sex and violence. The Family Life and Life Skills Education Program is a good support system for adolescents at the community level.

World Health Organization (WHO) has defined life skills as, "the abilities for adaptive and positive behavior that enable individuals to deal effectively with the demands and challenges of everyday life" (WHO, 1996).

UNICEF defines life skills as, "…a behavior change or behavior development approach designed to address a balance of three areas: Knowledge, attitude and skills…" Thus, life skills are essentially those abilities that help promote mental well-being and competence in young people as they face the realities of life.

The foundation on which the life skill approach is developed is drawn from various theories that have positively contributed to the growth and enrichment of life skill education. Social Learning Theory of Bandura (1977) is prominent among them. The other theories include child and adolescent development theory, cognitive problem-solving theory, social influence theory, multiple intelligence theory, problem behavior theory as well as risk and resilience theory (Mangrulkar, Whiteman, & Posner, 2001). From a cognitive behavioral viewpoint, the perception is that the life skills are the skills that are learnt or acquired and a person can be made conscious of its importance through training.

Life skills approach is an educational innovation that has spread in several countries since it was introduced in mid-1980's, thus showing its effectiveness. Comprehensive Life Skills Programs which developed in England, Canada, Australia and the United States have now spread to over 30 countries. In this country i.e. India, most of the initiatives have come from non-governmental organization sector besides some from the governmental sector (Yadav & Iqbal, 2009).

Developed by Dr. Botvin in the year 1984, a leading prevention expert, Life Skills Training is backed by over 20 scientific studies and is recognized as a Model or Exemplary Program by an array of government agencies, including the U.S. Department of Education and the Center for Substance Abuse Prevention.

Life Skills Training can be utilized in many context areas, issues, topics or subjects such as in prevention of drug abuse, sexual violence, teenage pregnancy, HIV/AIDS/STD prevention, suicide prevention, etc. However, UNICEF extends its use further into consumer education, environmental education, peace education or education for development, livelihood and income generation among others. In short, it empowers young people to take positive actions to protect themselves and to promote health and positive social relationships.

Life skills are essentially those abilities that help promote mental well-being and competence in young people as they face the challenges of life. Both UNICEF and WHO agree that life skills are generally applied in various aspects of life such as in the context of health and social events like human relationships, learning about social influences on behavior and learning about rights and responsibilities as well as being taught in the context of health problems (Yadav & Iqbal, 2009).

Life skills, thus, enable individuals to translate knowledge, attitudes and values into actual abilities i.e. what to do and how to do it. Life skills are abilities that enable individuals to behave in healthy ways given the desire to do so and given the scope and opportunity to do so. However, these are not a panacea. "How to do abilities" are not the only factors that affect behavior. If the model is placed within a larger and more comprehensive framework, there would be many factors that relate to the motivation and ability to behave in positive ways to prevent health problems. These factors include such things as social support, cultural and environment factors, etc.

Life skill acquisition facilitates a complete and integrated development of individuals to function effectively as social beings. Life skills can also be applied in the contexts of social and health events. With life skills, one is able to explore alternatives, weigh pros and cons and make rational decisions in solving each problem or issue as it arises. It also entails being able to establish productive interpersonal relationships with others. Developing life skills helps adolescents in translating knowledge, attitude and values into healthy behavior that makes their lives meaningful and fruitful. Life skills also help in empowering girls by developing healthy behavior/ practices and helping them to avoid risky behavior/ situations and to make appropriate decisions at the right time.

Life skill education aims to provide the adolescents with strategies to make healthy choices that contribute to a meaningful life. Life skills are the abilities that help to promote mental well being and competence in young people as they face the realities of life. It helps the young people to take positive actions to protect themselves and to promote healthy and meaningful social relationship.

Life Skills Model

Life skills have been defined as "Personal and social skills required for young people to function confidently and competently with themselves, with other people and with the wider community" (TACADE, 1990).

Hamburg (1990) defined life skills training as teaching of skills for survival, living with others and succeeding in a complex society. Nelson Jones (1993) states that life skills are personally responsible sequences of self-help choices in specific psychological skill areas conducive to mental wellness.

'Life skills are skills, strengths and capabilities that help individuals face problems of their everyday life with a positive attitude and go about with their everyday tasks effectively.' (Joseph, 2008). People require a repertoire of life skills according to their developmental tasks and to deal with specific problems of living (Bahrani, 2011).

Life skills are, thus, the skills necessary for successful living. They are the abilities for adaptive and positive behavior that enable individuals to deal with the demands and challenges of everyday living. Essential life skills include such things as being able to recognize and describe one's feeling, giving and receiving feedback, recognizing assumptions, setting realistic and attainable goals and employing problem-solving strategies. In other words, life skills are abilities that facilitate the physical, mental and emotional well-being of an individual and competence in young people as they face the realities of life.

Core Life Skills

During the 21st century, life globally is undergoing significant transition and changes. Today, more and more societal pressures, greater complexity, uncertainty and diversity, rapid changes in the environment and continued deprivation put adolescents at the crossroads of their lives facing an uncertain future in undertaking the responsibilities of adulthood and to enter the world of work. Among the most affected are the adolescents. Core life skills play an essential function for the adolescents who are the future of the country.

The study conducted by Khera and Khosla (2012) investigated the relationship between self-concept and core life skills of randomly selected 500 adolescents studying in secondary classes of Sarvodaya schools situated in South Delhi who had undergone for YUVA (LSP). The Major findings of the study revealed that there is a positive co-relation between Core Affective Life Skill and Self Concept of adolescents which means that those who possess these essential life skills have better confidence in all aspects.

Core life skills are, thus, the abilities for adaptive and positive behavior that enable individuals to deal effectively with the demands and challenges of everyday life. 'Adaptive' means that a person is flexible in approach and is able to adjust in different circumstances. 'Positive behavior' implies that a person is forward looking and even in difficult situations can find a ray of hope and opportunities to find solutions to the problematic situations. These core life skills can be categorized as under:

Classification of Core Life Skills

According to CBSE Teachers' Manual for Life Skills Education, Life skills are essentially those abilities that help promote mental well-being and competence in young people as they face the realities of life. These are generally applied in the context of health and social events. These are broadly classified under three domains, namely Cognitive skills, Affective skills and Psychomotor skills.

- **Cognitive Life Skills:** Cognitive life skills consist of six core life skills such as Self-awareness, Critical thinking, Decision making, Effective communication, Creative thinking and Problem solving.
- **Affective Life Skills:** Affective life skills consist of four core life skills such as Coping with stress, Empathy, Interpersonal relationship and Coping with emotions.
- **Psychomotor Life Skills:** Psychomotor life skills include physical skills such as movement, coordination, manipulation, dexterity, grace, strength, speed and finer motor skills.

Major Life Skills

WHO has identified the core life skills and provided them meaning accordingly. Based on the theoretical perspective i.e. Life skills are abilities for adaptive and positive behavior that enables individuals to deal effectively with demands and challenges of everyday life as well as various programs organized in different social settings, sets of ten core general life skills have been identified across each culture for promotion of psycho-social health of children and adolescents. These core life skills are decision making, problem solving, empathy, self-awareness, communication, inter personal relationships, coping with emotions, coping with stress, creative thinking and critical thinking.

Researches demonstrate that possessing life skills may be critical to young people's ability to positively adapt to and deal with the demands and challenges of life. Life Skill training is based on the philosophy that young people should be empowered to take more responsibility for their own actions (Vranda & Rao, 2011).

The set of core life skills which help in promoting health and well-being of children and adolescents include the following skills:

- Decision making
- Problem solving
- Creative thinking
- Critical thinking
- Effective communication
- Interpersonal relationship skills
- Self-awareness
- Empathy
- Coping with emotions
- Coping with stress
- **Decision Making:** The process of assessing an issue by considering all possible/available options and the effects those different decisions might have on them.
- **Problem Solving**: Having made the decisions about each of the options, choosing the one which suits the best, following it through even in the face impediments and going through the process again till a positive outcome of the problem is achieved.

- **Creative Thinking**: It is the ability to look beyond one's direct experiences and address issues. It contributes to both decision making and problem solving by enabling one to explore the available alternatives and various consequences of one's actions or non-action. It helps one to look beyond one's direct experiences and even if no problem is identified or no decision is to be made, creative thinking can help one to respond adaptively and with flexibility to the situations of one's daily life.
- **Critical Thinking**: It is an ability to analyze information and experiences in an objective manner. Critical thinking can contribute by helping one to recognize and assess the factors that influence attitudes and behavior such as values, peer pressure and the media.
- **Effective Communication**: Effective communication means that one is able to express oneself, both verbally and non-verbally, in ways that are appropriate to the cultures and situations. This means being able to express opinions, desires, needs and fears. It also means being able to ask for advice and help in a time of need.
- **Interpersonal Relationships**: Interpersonal relationship skills help one to relate in positive ways with the people one interacts with. This means being able to make and keep friendly relationships which can be of great importance to the mental and social well-being. It also includes keeping good relations with family members who are an important source of social support.
- **Self-Awareness:** Self-awareness includes recognition of oneself, the character, the strengths and weaknesses, the desires and dislikes. Developing self-awareness can help one to recognize when one is stressed or feels under pressure. It is also often a prerequisite for effective communication and interpersonal relations as well as for developing empathy for others.
- **Empathy:** Empathy is an ability to imagine what life is like for another person, even in a situation that one may not be familiar with. Empathy can help one to understand and accept others who may be very different from oneself which can improve social interactions, for example, in situations of ethnic or cultural diversity. Empathy can also help to encourage nurturing behavior towards people in need of care and assistance or tolerance, as is the case with HIV/AIDS sufferers or people with mental disorders who may be stigmatized and ostracized by the very people they depend upon for support.

- **Coping with Emotions:** Coping with emotions involves recognizing emotions in oneself and others, being aware of how emotions influence behavior and being able to respond to emotions appropriately. Intense emotions like anger or sorrow can have negative effects on one's health if one does not react appropriately.
- **Coping with Stress:** Coping with stress recognizes the sources of stress in one's life, recognizing how this affects one and acting in ways that help to control one's levels of stress. This means that one may take action to reduce the sources of stress, for example, by making changes to one's physical environment or lifestyle.

Inevitably, social and cultural factors determine the exact nature of these life skills. For example, eye contact may be encouraged in boys for effective communication but not for girls in some societies, so gender issues will arise in identifying the nature of life skills for psycho-social competence. The exact content of life skills education must therefore be determined at the country level or in a local context. However, described in general terms, life skills are being taught in such a wide variety of countries that they appear to have relevance across cultures.

While investigating into the awareness among primary and secondary school teachers towards population problem and attitudes towards population education, the study carried out by Agarwal (1990) revealed that caste seemed to be a significant variable in awareness of population problem and attitude towards the population education.

Abraham (1991) conducted a study on the awareness, attitudes and skills of secondary school students on population issues. It was found that a significant role is being played by religion, sex and educational background of father and mother towards knowledge on population issues.

Need of Life Skills Education for Adolescents

Adolescence is the most critical phase in the life of an individual. It denotes the transitional stage from childhood to adulthood marked by conspicuous physical, cognitive, emotional and social changes. The inbuilt taboos existing in the society in the form of control and support from the near and dear ones guide the adolescents to grow into a mature adult.

However, life styles have changed due to globalization and technology invasion in day to day affairs in a big way. The highly competitive world of today and the absence of traditional norms and support have heightened the level of stress among adolescents, thus resulting in multiple mental health issues such as depression, anxiety, loneliness, rejection, diffidence, anger, confliction in interpersonal relationship and failures (Smith, 2004).

Understanding the need to equip children with life skills, schools have expressed a need to develop life skills education programs as part of curriculum at different levels of schooling process. Education plays an important role towards the overall development of human beings. Life skill education through school education helps in the development of a sound personality of the child.

According to a Program on Mental Health, Life Skills Education in Schools, Division of Mental Health and Prevention of Substance Abuse, World Health Organization (1994), Life skills Education Programs in schools are important because of the following reasons:

Firstly, psycho-social competence is a person's ability to deal effectively with the demands and challenges of everyday life. It is a person's ability to maintain a state of mental well-being and to demonstrate this in their adaptive and positive behavior while interacting with others, with the culture and the environment.

Secondly, psycho-social competence has an important role to play in the promotion of health in its broadest sense; in terms of physical, mental and social well-being. In particular, where health problems are related to behavior and where the behavior is related to an inability to deal effectively with stresses and pressures in life, the enhancement of psycho-social competence could make an important contribution.

Thirdly, schools are the places where an individual gets opportunities to interact with people from different social strata, values, traditions and beliefs. This is the place where a person learns about the norms of the society. If awareness about concept of life skills is provided in an integrated manner to the young students in schools, it will help them to deal with complex social situations in later life with required maturity and composure. Therefore, the need to take up these concepts of life skill education in schools is thought of and implemented in the form of life skills education in schools.

Life Skills Education in Schools

The need and importance for school-based life skill education programs has been reflected in its inclusion in the school curricula by NCERT and CBSC. Majority of the schools in India focus on development of scholastic, reading and writing skills of the children. They feel that improvement in marks of the students will increase their school's reputation, as well as the confidence and personality of their students. The curricula are mostly lacking focus on the transitional age of adolescents which has significant impact in the life of students. The schools are not able to satisfy their psycho-social needs, unable to communicate with others, inability to identify risk factors, unable to make good decisions and finally ended up in frequent failures and suicidal attempts by the adolescents. Lack of knowledge and awareness of parents about the concerns of growing children complicates the problem further.

According to the Central Board of Secondary Education (CBSE) Manual for Teachers on Life Skills Education, adolescence is a critical period for the development of self-identity. The process of acquiring a sense of self is linked to physiological changes and also learning to negotiate the social and psychological demands of being young adults. Responsible handling of issues like independence, intimacy and peer group dependence are concerns that need to be recognized and appropriate support needs to be given to cope with them.

In India, Central Board of Secondary Education (CBSE), after eight years of research, introduced "Continuous and Comprehensive Evaluation (CCE)" in IX and X class during the year 2010 with the grading system. The CCE is school based evaluation of students that covers all aspects of student's development. The evaluation and assessment are based on various areas as described in CBSE Teacher's Manual in three parts; where part-2 consists of co-scholastic area in two parts: Medium or Format and Adapt (remix, transform and build upon the material) under the attribution non-commercial terms.

Sharma (2003) had published a paper on measuring life skills of adolescents in a secondary school at Kathmandu, Nepal. The objective of this study was to develop a scale to measure life skills and to assess the levels of life skills among adolescents of a secondary school. She concluded that most of the teachers were not aware of the concept of life skills. Maternal education was significantly associated with higher life skill levels among adolescents. Connectedness and family support were other important factors influencing the level of life skills among adolescents.

Gamble (2006), in his article on teaching life skills for student's success, had written that Chicago Public Schools (CPS) had recognized that their graduates were still struggling to find employment. The study also concluded that those graduates who found employment were having difficulty in retaining their jobs. Chicago educators hired the company. All Students learnt to write Curriculum Vitae that address employability skills for junior high school students, university students and adults entering the workforce. This article also describes teachers and student's responses toward the project. Chicago Public Schools then piloted this project with great success.

In an article by Jones et al. (2006) titled 'Developing an Entrepreneurial Life Skills Summer School' in which it was said that successive governments in United Kingdom have increasingly stressed the need for a more enterprising society. Much of the emphasis had been placed upon educationists to introduce more elements of enterprise into the school curriculum at all levels for which new and innovative ways to initiate the subject matter were increasingly being sought. This article described a summer school that was a part of this initiative. It was stressed that there was a difference between Traditional and Enterprise modes of learning. It also contested that as compared to traditional methods of teaching and learning; enterprise education required a different pedagogical approach and aimed to qualitatively change the educational experiences. It was suggested that traditional teaching was better suited to the needs of the "old" economy while the enterprising approach was more conducive to the needs of the "new" flexible market economy.

Lineo (2009) had conducted a study on life skill education of adolescents. The introduction of life skill education at both basic and tertiary levels was meant among other things to improve all aspects of the quality education, thereby ensuring equitable access to appropriate learning and facilitating Education for All (EFA) and Millennium Development Goals (MDG) initiatives. The purpose was to explore the main components of life skill education programs in place of Lesotho education system to address developmental problems such as poverty reduction, preventing spread of HIV/AIDS as well as alcohol and drug abuse. The study examined how the life skill education programs were implemented and evaluated at Primary schools, Secondary schools and institutions of Higher Learning. Qualitative data was collected through document review and analysis; interviews of policy-makers in the Ministry of Education and Training, Deans of the Faculty of Education in the institutions of Higher Learning, principals, education officers and curriculum developers. The findings highlighted a number of issues and potentials emanating from assessment and evaluation as well as quality and teacher capacity in the delivery of the programs. In order to fully address the issues of equity and access of essential life skills, the study recommended that the government of Lesotho should also consider for delivering the programs through Open and Distance Learning mode and to learners participating in Open and Distance Learning.

Khanna and Sharma (2014) conducted a study to understand the role of engaging youth in a creative activity like puppetry in enhancing the life skills of youth and to assess its potential as a medium of edutainment. A sample of

32 postgraduate women students participated in puppetry workshop with focus on selected health issues and an equal number of 32 students formed the non-participant group. Findings of this study revealed that mean score of several life skills were significantly higher for the participant group as compared to that of non-participant group as well as than the National Norms. The study concluded that life skills of youth can be significantly enhanced by engaging them in creative and participatory group assignments like puppetry. It was also concluded that engaging youth in puppetry could be used as an effective teaching learning method and for enhancing their life skills.

Bardhan (2016) has made an attempt to understand whether and how school children learnt life skills through their continuous involvement with school authorities, their classmates and counselors and its impact on modifying their behaviour. The study was conducted among the school children with high risk behaviour. Along with children, life skill education intervention was carried out for their parents also. Qualitative methodology was adopted for the research study. Data was collected through case studies. Meta-analysis of case-studies was done to assess the impact of life skill education intervention in bringing out behavioral changes among children. The study proved that continuous life skill training along with structured counseling helped in developing positive changes among children with problem behaviour. It also helped children to develop friendly relationship with their teachers, peers and parents.

Various skills like leadership, responsibility, communication, intellectual capacity, self-esteem, interpersonal skill etc. extend to its maximum level if these are practiced effectively. There is an essential need to create life skill education program as the cornerstone of various youth programs and an integral part of the formal education process.

Today's formal education system is lopsided as it provides more of knowledge related concepts rather than skills, attitude and value-oriented education. Looking into the needs of present day complicated life, one needs more than that of simple knowledge. Knowledge which is not put to practical application is of no use. One needs more of skills to put the knowledge into use to lead a meaningful and successful life.

Reports of various commissions and committees on education have pointed towards the lack of emphasis on training aspect as well as process aspect in the present-day education system. Developing these skills needs to occupy an important aspect in the teaching learning process. These skills are of varied nature like soft skills, communication skills, techno-savvy skills, info-savvy skills, techno-pedagogy skills, spiritual skills, research skills and life skills at large.

Life skill learning is facilitated by use of participatory learning approach; peer supported learning and practical community development projects. It is not only an active process, but it must also include experiential learning i.e. practical experience and the reinforcement of skills for each adolescent in a supportive learning environment. Life skills education is a dynamics and evolving process which must involve children, parents and the local community in making decisions regarding the content of the program.

In life skill education program, children are actively involved in a dynamic teaching and learning process. Various methods used to facilitate this active involvement of children in the teaching learning process include working in small groups and pairs, brain storming, role play, games, debates and so on.

A life skill lesson may start with a teacher exploring with the students what their ideas or knowledge is about a particular situation in which a life skill can be used. The children may be asked to discuss the issues raised in more detail in small groups or with a partner. They may then engage in short role play scenarios or take part in activities that allow them to practice the skill in different situations as the actual practice of a skill is a vital component of life skill education. Finally, the teacher assigns homework to encourage the children to further discuss and practice the skill with their families and friends.

Life Skill Education Approach

Adolescence is a period when the physical, intellectual and all other capabilities are very high, but their anti-social activities and behavior are deteriorating all their capabilities. Hence, they become a burden on the society. Imparting life skill training for inculcating life skills helps the adolescents to overcome such difficulties in their lives. Core life skills play an essential part of adolescent's development who are the future of the country.

Life skill education is a value-added program which aims to provide adolescents with strategies to make healthy choices that contribute to a meaningful life. It helps them to understand their self and to assess their skills, abilities and areas of development. It also helps the adolescents to get along with other people and adjust with their environment and in making responsible decisions. The main objective of life skill education is to enable the learner to develop a concept of oneself as a person of worth and dignity. Life skill education is, thus, a basic learning need for all adolescents.

Skill based approach in life skill education follows well established mentoring techniques to develop student's innate qualities and also motivates them to adopt socially acceptable pattern of life style particularly, strategy consisting of a group of people combined together to help themselves by identifying their talents and directing them to choose appropriate steps to enhance their skills and abilities as part of their development.

Life Skill approach is a fine interactive educational methodology which focuses on more than just information but to develop or change attitude and behavior/ practices. The psychological push factors such as inability to tackle emotional pain, conflicts, frustrations and anxieties about the future are often the driving forces for high risk behavior.

UNESCO with the Ministry of Human Resource and Development organized a workshop on life skill education in December 1998. The basic purpose of this workshop was to look for a life skill approach that can be integrated with the Non-Formal Education curriculum so that the out-of-school children can manage the day to day situations in their lives. The program was developed keeping the goals in mind i.e. to involve the staff, parents, peer group and community to help the out-of-school children develop positive qualities, to ensure that the young ones are committed positively to their families, to help them solve problems co-operatively, to allow the learners to handle negative pressures from their peers. It was discussed in the workshop that life skills should not be taught in isolation but should be integrated with health and other major life issues education. The main conclusion of the workshop was that everybody needs life skill education and the programs should be developed to integrate the life skill education with the Non-Formal Education curriculum.

Life Skill Education for adolescents is aimed at facilitating the development of psycho-social skills that are required to deal with the demands and challenges of everyday life. Life Skill Education should be designed to facilitate the practice and reinforcement of life skills in culturally and developmentally appropriate way. It contributes to the promotion of personal and social development, prevention of health and social problems and protection of human rights. Life Skill Education enables individuals to translate knowledge, attitudes and values into actual abilities, thus enabling them to behave in a healthy way.

Botvin et al. (1980) conducted a study on preventing the onset of cigarette smoking through life skill training. The effectiveness of 10-sessions of psycho-social life skill approach in the prevention of cigarette smoking was tested on 8th, 9th, and 10th graders in New York. The program was designed to address both the social and psychological factors promoting the onset of smoking by attempting to: a) increase student's ability to cope with direct pressures to smoke; b) decrease their susceptibility to indirect pro-smoking social influences and; c) improve their ability to cope with anxiety. The program was conducted by allied health professionals and utilized methods of group discussion, modeling and behavior rehearsal. Results of this study indicated significant differences between the experimental and control groups in terms of the proportion of new "experimental smokers", Furthermore, there were significantly greater post-test changes for the experimental group on several of the knowledge and psychological measures, thereby suggesting that the decrease in the onset of smoking behavior among the experimental subjects did occur for the hypothesized reasons.

Botvin and Baker (1984) conducted a study on substance abuse prevention. The prevention strategy attempted to reduce intra-personal pressure to smoke, drink excessively or use marijuana by fostering the development of general life skills as well as teaching student's tactics for resisting direct inter-personal pressure to use these substances. Result of the study indicated that the prevention program had a significant impact on cigarette smoking, excessive drinking and marijuana use when implemented by peer leaders. Furthermore, significant changes were also evident with respect to selected cognitive, attitudinal and personality predisposing variables in a direction consistent with non-substance use. These results provided further support for the efficacy of broad-spectrum smoking prevention strategy and tentative support for its applicability for the prevention of other forms of substance abuse.

The reason for getting such results could be summarized in this way. Life skills applied to drug/substance use prevention are supposed to facilitate the practice and reinforcement of psycho-social skills that contribute to the promotion of personal and social development such as self-awareness, empathy, communication skills, interpersonal skills, creative thinking, critical thinking, coping with emotions and coping with stress. Empathy and interpersonal sensitivity may be turned simply into useful 'tools' for adjusting delinquent or disturbed young people to schooling. Lack of empathic concern, poor communicative responsiveness and high emotional contagion significantly contributed to reduced personal accomplishment (O'Donnell, Stueve, Doval, Duran, Haber, Atnafou, Johnson, Grant, Murray, Juhn, Tang, & Piessens, 1999).

Implementation of Life Skill Education

In order to have an effective implementation of life skill education, there is a need for professionally trained and skilled personnel. Professional training requires a purposely planned program of study prepared by experts/ teachers with favorable attitude which have the approval of a competent authority and a group of experts to train the trainers of life skills education.

The Department of Adult and Continuing Education (2006) organized an International Workshop on Life Skill Education for Youth Development in the University of Madras in India. The workshop was organized with the support of the University Grants Commission, New Delhi. The main points discussed in the workshop were that life skills are essentially those activities that help promote mental well-being and competence in young people as they face the realities of life. Developing life skills helps adolescents translate knowledge, attitude and values into healthy behaviors that improve their lives in general. The objectives of the workshop were to integrate Life Skill Education in the curriculum at the college level, to design and develop training manual on Life Skill Education, to design and develop learning modules for Life Skill Education, to design and develop training methods and programs for the colleges and the community at large.

Kaur and Kaur (2014) studied the attitude of prospective teachers towards life skill education using descriptive survey method. Data was collected from 200 prospective teachers of Patiala district of Punjab, India who were selected by stratified sampling technique by employing life skill opinion questionnaire (NIMHANS) and self-prepared background information sheet. Percentage analysis and chi-square test were used to analyze the data. The findings revealed that there were significant gender and location-wise differences in the attitude of teacher trainees towards life skill education.

Adolescence is a period of mental development as well when young adolescents are receptive fast learners, capable of integrating new knowledge and hungry for its application into their rapidly changing lives. Additionally, with the obvious changes occurring in their bodies, adolescents are receptive to new knowledge about reproduction, health and nutrition. Even for those who have dropped out of formal schooling, literacy can be rapidly attained and valuable information to "The Facts for Life" can be more readily transmitted and assimilated at this age than at any other period of life.

However, it is probably not the formal education and knowledge alone that accounts for the remarkable effect of education on health and well-being of adolescents. Literacy grants power and status to young adolescents themselves as well as the people they live with. The socialization process enables them to gain self-esteem and develop relationships that will provide continuing information, knowledge and wisdom in the years ahead. Schooling provides a unique opportunity for adolescents to develop a new image for each other and break down the age old prejudices, which are responsible for extreme gender disparity characterizing much of the Indian Society.

Still, there are many opportunities alive in India today that could transform the psychological and social scene within few years. First, of course, is the formal education of adolescents. Self-esteem and value in the eyes of society are best engendered during this period and will have long term benefits to overall efforts, not only in health but also in environment, economics and the community life. Young adolescents gain access to new sources of information and knowledge and begin to take a mature and positive role in their own communities.

An attempt has been made by the author in this research to understand the impact of life skill intervention program in modifying the attitude and behavior/ practices of adolescents and how it enabled them to lead a healthy and positive life. The researcher had conducted a series of training sessions with the target group population and imparted them life skill education required to solve their problems and observed how it enabled them to overcome the difficult situations (Nanda, 2001).

The findings of research carried out by the author aiming to find out the impact of Nutrition, Health, Hygiene and Child Care (NHHCC) Education program on Knowledge, Attitudes and Practices/ Behavior (KAP/KAB) of adolescents revealed a highly significant improvement in knowledge scores of adolescent girls as a result of NHHCC education, the quantum of improvement being 2.0-2.4 fold. As attitudes are affected by knowledge, a highly significant improvement in attitude scores was also observed to the tune of 1.5-1.6 fold. However, the change in attitudes was more in younger girls as compared to older ones. Surprisingly, very highly significant improvement in scores of practices to the tune of 9.9 fold in younger and 4.3 fold in older adolescent girls was observed as a result of improved knowledge, which is evident from a significantly positive correlation between knowledge and practices ($r = 0.49$) (Nanda, 2001). The participatory methods used during the educational intervention facilitated change in practices/ behavior of adolescents by enabling them to feel more confident, practice through target behavior and experience their reinforcing value, as advocated by Social Learning Theory of Bandura (1977).

Attitudes are dispositions of a person to react in a certain manner towards a situation or an idea. These are formed on the basis of direct or indirect experiences, which a person gains while dealing with the problems, one has to face in a particular situation. Hence, need satisfaction of persons forms the basis of positive attitudes and vice-versa. Since knowledge gained by a person helps in satisfying one's needs, the areas of sound knowledge become the basis for positive attitudes and vice-versa. Further, attitudes are strengthened through persuasive communication, resulting in formation of desirable behavior. However, the conservative attitude of parents and the society due to socio-cultural backwardness worked as negative forces, thus limiting the scope of much improvement in attitude scores of these adolescent girls in the present study (Nanda, 2001).

The findings of this research have been supported by a highly significant correlation between knowledge and practices/ behavior but non-significant correlation between attitudes and practices. These findings are based on the assumption that higher knowledge results in better practices and vice-versa. Correct knowledge is a pre-requisite in acquiring and changing beliefs in the right direction. With correct beliefs coupled with continued persuasion, practices also change; though take longer time to do so. One may not always be able to put into practice, what one knows and believes to be correct because of variety of social, environmental and cultural factors which may hinder in putting knowledge into practice. A significantly positive correlation between knowledge and attitude suggests that knowledge inspires confidence and improves attitudes, although attitudes are difficult to change (Nanda, 2001).

An interesting finding that came to light in this research was that learning by younger adolescents was better as compared to older ones in all aspects of knowledge, attitudes and practices/behavior. Though learning is a continuing life long process but the likely reasons for better learning response by younger adolescents was that they were more receptive because of their impressionable minds, had less of negative learning from the environment, lesser distraction of minds, thus enabling them to concentrate more and attend to learning activities, lesser responsibility and more flexibility in their attitudes and beliefs. Moreover, participatory approach and interactive methods proved useful in significantly improving their knowledge, changing attitudes and correcting the wrong practices (Nanda, 2001).

The results of the study conducted by Budhani and Singh (1996) on communication support for training rural youth in 'TRYSEM" as a component of Integrated Rural Development Program (IRDP) also revealed that younger adolescents gained more knowledge than older ones, when exposed to the messages through combination of media. It is, therefore, much easier to bring about a desirable change in knowledge, attitudes and practices of young adolescents, who can serve as a potential agent of change for bringing about an improvement in their own nutritional status as well as the nutritional status of the community.

Effectiveness of Life Skills Education Program

Many studies have confirmed the effectiveness of life skills training programs on high-risk behavior, the ability to cope with the pressures and development of psychological variables.

Zollinger et al. (2003) conducted a study on evaluation of school-based tobacco prevention and control programs which yielded mixed results. This study assessed the impact of the Life Skill Training Curriculum on middle school student's knowledge, attitude and ability to make good lifestyle decisions in Marion Country. During the years 1997 to 2000, students in grades six to eight in the study schools received the Life Skill Training Curriculum. Survey data was used to compare tobacco use behavior, attitudes and knowledge of those exposed to and those not exposed to the program. Of the students surveyed, 12.5 percent were currently smoking. There were significantly fewer current smokers and more students who were exposed to the program indicated that they intended to stay smoke-free. Fewer of those students participating in the program "hung out" with smokers and many students told that they should easily refuse a cigarette if offered one. Students completing the Life Skill Teaching Curriculum were more knowledgeable about the harmful effects of smoking. Program effects were different for male and female students as well as for White and Black students.

Botvin et al. (2003) examined the effectiveness of Substance Abuse Prevention Program in preventing tobacco and alcohol use among elementary school students in grades 3 to 6. The Substance Abuse Prevention Program teaches social resistance skills as well as general personal and social competence skills. Rates of substance abuse behavior, attitudes, knowledge, normative expectations and related variables were examined among students (N= 1090) from 20 schools who were randomly assigned to either receive the prevention program (9 schools, n= 426) or serve as a control group (11 schools, n= 664) who did not receive the prevention program. Data were analyzed at both the individual-level and school-level.

Sherman et al. (2009) performed a study to evaluate the effectiveness of interventions in the form of life skill training and peer network training on reducing substance abuse behavior and inappropriate sexual behavior in adolescents suffering from meta-amphetamines abuse. The results confirmed a reduction in methamphetamine use, improvement in appropriate sexual behavior and reduced sexually transmitted infections.

Poobalan et al. (2009) conducted a review of reviews to identify characteristics of effective sex and relationship education (SRE) interventions and/or programs in young people to improve sexual health and identify barriers and facilitators for the implementation of the same. Six bibliographic databases were searched from 1986 to 2006 for systematic reviews that assessed SRE interventions or programs in participants between 10 and 18 years old and their partners. All outcomes of improvement in sexual health were assessed and 30 systematic reviews were included. Effective interventions and/or programs tended to be those targeting younger age groups before they become sexually active, focused interventions tailored to the physical and biological development stages, theory based, and abstinence education programs that incorporate values of relationships and provide skills training and links to contraceptive services. Adequate training of personnel delivering the interventions and culturally sensitive programs were identified as important facilitators of effectiveness of SRE programs/ interventions.

Manocha (2013) conducted a study with the purpose of investigating the effect of training on the development of undergraduate female students, aged 18 to 21 years, from Panchkula, Haryana in India. Impact analysis of training program was carried out in terms of gain in knowledge index in the respective fields for improving the health and hygiene status of beneficiaries, training on diseases and vaccination, yoga and meditation, reproductive health and drug addiction. Results of the study revealed that the knowledge index improved from a score of 17.37 at pre-test to 20.80 at post-test. Components of Skills index enhanced by 4.5 points and personality index improved from 42.07 to 48.91 after the training program. The study concluded that training programs are powerful medium for skill acquisition and capacity building of adolescent girls.

A study was conducted by Sikandra and Kumar (2014) on 160 mothers of school children, ages 9 to 15 years, who were selected randomly from Hisar and Gurugram in Haryana, India. In this study, nutritional knowledge of obese respondents was assessed using self-developed questionnaire both before and after imparting nutrition education to the parents of the respondents. Findings of the study revealed that majority of the parents had low level of knowledge about various aspects of nutrition before the exposure to nutrition education program. The mean score of knowledge improved significantly to medium or high level after imparting nutrition education to the parents in both the cities of Haryana.

Choudhary et al. (2014) studied the impact of visual media regarding nutrition messages given to 120 school children, including both boys and girls, studying in 9th and 10th class. Regarding almost all messages, knowledge of respondents was below median at pre-exposure stage which improved to above median at post-exposure stage. Pre- and post-exposure scores indicated a significant gain in knowledge and change in attitude for most of the messages. However, practice change was still quite slow as change in habit is a slow process and requires continuous efforts which most likely lead to a positive eating behavior.

Nutrition Education, as one of the required dimensions of Life Skill Education, has been emphasized by Sindhu et al. (2014) who opined that young vulnerable minds of today are exposed to high sugar, high fat, high sodium, low fiber junk food on one hand and to the glamour world of fashion through the media on the other hand, thus resulting in a mix of obese or undernourished youth with a very low population which is nutritionally healthy. Thus, nutrition education, as a part of life skill education, would be an efficacious tool for empowering the youth to act responsibly, take initiative and take control of their lives.

Another study by Sangwan et al. (2014) focused on strengthening knowledge towards family life education among rural youth of Haryana in India with the objective to assess the existing knowledge of rural youth regarding family life as well as to develop and implement family life education program for enhancing knowledge. Various aspects of family living i.e. personal hygiene, nutrition and health, gender sensitivity, family planning, maternal and child care, HIV/AIDS and physical and emotional health were assessed. The findings of the study revealed that majority of the respondents had low knowledge on all aspects of family life. However, their knowledge was strengthened by continuous personal contact programs, community-based programs and the use of audio-visual aids. Researchers recommended that imparting family life education should be made compulsory and regular feature at middle and high school level, especially for adolescent girls.

In the light of above discussion, it can be said that life skill training can specifically address the needs of children and adolescents growing up in disadvantaged environments that lack opportunities to develop these skills.

Health promotion and prevention programs focusing only on the transfer of information is less effective than programs incorporating skill development.

Life skills, thus, include psycho-social competencies and interpersonal skills that help adolescents to make informed decisions, solve problems, think critically and creatively, communicate effectively, build healthy relationships, empathize with others and cope with managing their lives in a healthy and productive manner.

Life Skills and Self Esteem

The self-esteem of an adolescent is an important contributor to his growth and helps him in dealing with the difficulties. Studies have found that one third to one-half of adolescents struggle with low self-esteem, especially in early adolescence (Harter, 1990; Hirsch & Dubois, 1991). The results of low self-esteem can be temporary but in serious cases can lead to various problems, including depression, delinquency, self-inflicted injuries, suicide (Battle, 1990; Bhatti, 1992) and anorexia nervosa. Miller (1988) demonstrated that a program to increase self-esteem which significantly changed the attitudes of students regarding their alcohol and drug use.

Researches have shown that high self-esteem can help adolescents with positive focus and happiness, thereby increasing the likelihood to be more successful in career and relationships. On the other hand, Trzesniewski et al. (2006) found that low self-esteem during adolescence predicts poor mental health, worse economic well-being and higher level of criminal activity in young adulthood. Imparting life skill education to children and adolescents will bring valuable benefits which include promotion of self-esteem, inner peace, self-confidence etc. (TACADE, 1990).

Life skills education is suggested by many as a prevention and development approach to improve the level of self-esteem. On adolescent students, Maryam and her colleagues (2011) in their investigation to find out the effectiveness of life skill training on adolescent students found that life skill training led to a significant increase in self-esteem of the study group. The researchers concluded that mental health programs such as life skills training can decline school and educational problems. Life skill education can promote social adjustment (Rahmati, Adibrad, Tahmasian, & Sedghpour, 2010); anger control (Feindler, Ecton, Kingsley, & Dubey, 1986); enhanced self-esteem (Young, Kelley, & Denny, 1997) and an improvement in academic performance, as reported in various researches that evaluated the effectiveness of life skill education.

The aim of the study conducted by Yadav and Iqbal (2009) was to see the impact of life skill training on self-esteem, adjustment and empathy among adolescents. Total sample comprised of 60 students (30 males and 30 females) from Delhi in India who had received life skill training from the team of Expressions India. Self Esteem Inventory (school form), Adjustment Inventory for School Students (AISS) and the Empathy Quotient (EQ) were administered in a group session one by one in two or three days both before training were given and after the training. In the post condition, test scores were obtained after 5 months of training. The result showed that subjects improved significantly in post condition on self-esteem, emotional adjustment, educational adjustment, total adjustment and empathy. However, no significant difference was found on social adjustment in pre and post conditions. Overall training was very effective as subjects improved in the post condition on all measures except one, thus showing that Life skill training do show positive results in bringing change in adolescent's attitude, thought and behavior by providing supportive environment to them.

The results of all these studies clearly illustrate the positive effect of life skills training to adolescents and importance of self-esteem as an important personality variable that needs to be strengthened as it is directly related to negative behavior. If adolescents develop some life skills, then positive feelings of self-worth will follow or if such youth have positive feelings of self-worth, they will be more likely to develop and practice new life skills. It can be said that group learning provides opportunity for social skills by encouraging social interaction and thus promotes self-esteem in the subjects.

Life Skills and Mental Health

Mental health is defined as the adjustment of an individual to the world and to each other with maximum of effectiveness and happiness. It is the ability to maintain an even temper, an alert intelligence and a socially considerable behavior. Mentally healthy individuals have adequate self-acceptance, hold a realistic view of himself, enjoys freedom from inner conflicts and anxiety and possesses adequate adjustment within himself in terms of his deeds and thoughts to the best of his ability and suitably reacts with the environment in an intelligent way.

Mental health is a self-attitude that leads to a sense of identity, growth, development and self-actualization including investment in living, integrating and resistance to stress, autonomy, inner regulation and independence, preparation of reality without distortion and an environmental mastery with successful problem solving.

Mental health is thus a complex state of being, a sense of confidence in oneself and one's world. A mentally healthy person is able to see and gradually deal with the reality concerning himself and the world to relate to other people in ways that are satisfying both to him and to them, to accept and control his impulses and to learn and apply what he has learned. A mentally healthy person continues to grow throughout his life time building an earlier foundation of strength and flexibility as he meets the new tasks and situations. Life skills are the abilities that help to promote mental well-being and competence in young people as they face the realities of life.

A study conducted by Ramesht and Farshad (2010) on a sample of 500 students concluded that life skill training proved to be effective in increasing physical and mental health and also in decreasing the behavioural and social problems. Improvement in interpersonal relationship and reduction in aggression and behavioural problems were found among the participants who had attended a coping life skill training program (Sukhodolsky, Golub, Stone, & Orban, 2004).

The aim of the study by Nasser Sobhi-Gharamaleki and Soran Rajabi (2010) was to assess to effect of providing life skill training on mental health and self-esteem of university students. The study method was experimental research method. The type of design was before and after test design with control group. Statistical society of the present study comprised of all boys' students studying at University of Mohaghegh, Ardabili during the year 2009. Also, this study was conducted only on the individuals who gained 28 or more in DASS questionnaire (which evaluates three subscales of anxiety, depression, and stress) (n=210). At the next stage, the needed sample (i.e. 40 boy students i.e. 20 individuals in control group and 20 individuals in experimental group) was selected randomly and distributed in two mentioned groups randomly. Then, life skills were taught to the subjects of experimental group for 8 sessions in four weeks and the subjects of control group were exposed to no variable during this period. At the end, 3 individuals from experimental group were omitted; finally, the achieved data from 37 individuals was analyzed by descriptive statistics methods (frequency and percentage) as well as inferential statistics methods (independent t-test, MANOVA). The results showed that life skill training effects on decreasing mental disorders symptoms especially anxiety, depression and stress of students suspected to the mental disorder. This study showed that life skill training is a good method in decreasing mental disorders symptoms among the students.

Duhan and Aneja (2014) studied the life skills for lifetime through educational programme on a sample of 150 adolescent girls, aged 13 to 19 years, selected randomly from five selected villages of Hisar district, Haryana in India. Results of the study highlighted that during pre-testing, the highest percentage of adolescent girls were in medium category of stress followed by 32.6% girls in high level of stress. Further, results showed medium level of empathy among more than 50% of girls and an equal number of girls were having medium and high level of problem-solving skills. For creative and critical thinking aspect, maximum respondents were having medium level of thinking abilities. Post-test results revealed a significant improvement in almost all the life skill aspects. The study concluded that continuous life skill education is an important measure to improve the skills required to lead a good quality of life.

Katyal (2014) carried out an investigation aiming to get an insight into the resilience among adolescents, aged 13 to17 years, living in slum areas of Chandigarh in India and to find out the gender differences, if any, in their resilience. A sample of 100 adolescents, 50 boys and 50 girls, who were not receiving any formal education, was selected from four randomly selected slum areas of Chandigarh. The findings revealed that slum adolescents had moderate level of resilience. Majority of boys had moderate followed by low level of resilience whereas majority of girls had moderate followed by high level of resilience. Results of the study revealed significant gender differences in their resilience level.

This research undertaken by Jamali et al. (2016) aimed to study the effect of life skill training on mental health of Iranian middle school students. This experimental study was conducted in the year 2015 on 100 students in the city of Ghaemshahr (North of Iran), who were randomly selected and divided into two equal groups of intervention (n = 50) and control (n = 50). Qualified trainers provided eight sessions (two sessions a week for 2 hours) of life skills training to the intervention group for one month. The control group did not participate in any training sessions during the same period. Mental health of the participants in both groups was assessed by a questionnaire at pre- and post-training. Data were analyzed using descriptive and inferential (ANCOVA and paired t-test) statistical tests. Results of the study revealed that the average age of the participants in both groups was 13.5±1.01. ANCOVA test results revealed that the difference in average scores of violence, addiction, stress and sensation-seeking before and after the training was statistically significant in the intervention group and control groups ($p<0.001$). It can be concluded that Life skill training had positive effect on mental health of the participants. Given the importance of mental health in modern societies, it is necessary for schools to incorporate life skills in their curriculum to support the mental health of adolescents.

In conclusion, the results of these studies can be used to help in the improvement of the students' mental health and their ability to deal with inappropriate conditions. Hence, it is suggested that life skills training, as one of the most important educational issues, must be paid more attention to and also the students' mental health and emotional intelligence can be improved by continuing this education along with holding counseling sessions on students' problems.

Life Skills and Emotional Intelligence

Emotional intelligence is positively associated with acquiring life skills. Emotional intelligence is the ability to identify, use, understand and manage emotions in a positive way to relieve stress, communicate effectively, empathize with others, overcome challenges and diffuse conflict.

Emotional intelligence is an aggregate of individual's cognition of own and other's emotions, feeling, interpretation and action as per the environmental demand to manipulate the consequence which, in turn, result in superior performance and better human relationships.

Emotional intelligence is, thus, a measure of the degree to which a person makes use of his/her reasoning in the process of emotional responses (both positive and negative) in a given situation. Two types of emotional intelligence models are available in the existing literature: (a) Ability Model, which focuses on the mental abilities to define emotional and intelligence and; (b) Mixed Model which seeks to define emotional intelligence as a mixture of abilities and some personality traits and characteristics (Bhattacharya & Sengupta, 2007).

The most popular and accepted mixed model of emotional intelligence is the one proposed by Goleman (1995). He viewed emotional intelligence as a total of personal and social competencies. Personal competence determines how we manage ourselves whereas social competence determines how we handle our inter-personal relationships. In the later version of emotional intelligence model, Goleman (2001) proposed four components of emotional intelligence: Self-awareness, Self-management, Social awareness and Relationship Management. Goleman's (1995, 2001) model of emotional intelligence was based on the 'theory of performance'.

Emotional intelligence is, therefore, essentially required for adolescents as without intelligent guidance of emotions, they cannot respond to situations very flexibly, take advantage of the right time and right pace, make sense of ambiguous and contradictory messages, recognize the importance of different elements of a situation, find similarities between situations despite differences that may separate them, draw distinction between situations despite similarities that may link them, synthesize new concepts by taking old concepts and combining in new ways or develop ideas that are novel.

In this regard, Bastian et al. (2005) conducted a study on 246 first-year students to find out the relationship between emotional intelligence and having life skills. These life skills included life satisfaction, problem-solving and coping with stress. The results of the study revealed that emotional intelligence was significantly associated with the skills of life satisfaction, problem-solving and coping with stress. The relationship between emotional intelligence and life skills showed that higher emotional intelligence was significantly correlated with higher life satisfaction (r= 0.51), coping with stress (r= 0.36) and problem-solving (r= 0.55) and lower stress (r= 0.25).

Wong et al. (2007) indicated the need to have interventional researches on determining the effectiveness of training programs on promoting the level of emotional intelligence and the necessity of studies with cases and controls to compare the levels of emotional intelligence before and after training program.

The study carried out by Lolaty et al. (2012) aimed at determining the effect of life skill training on the emotional intelligence among the first-year students of Mazandaran University of Medical Sciences. In this experimental study, the subjects were selected by random sampling and allocated into two groups: Case group (n=20) and control group (n=19); the two groups were matched for gender, experience of stressful life events in the past six months, level of interest in the field of study and level of emotional intelligence. The two groups responded to Bar-on Emotional Quotient Inventory before starting the experiment. Subsequently, the case group underwent life skill training. After the training, Bar-on Emotional Quotient Inventory was responded by the case and control groups again. The data was analyzed using descriptive statistics including Chi-square test, paired and independent t-tests, using SPSS software version 15. Results of the study revealed that in the case group, the scores of emotional intelligence after life skill training were significantly improved (t= 11.703 df= 19 P= 0.001) while no significant difference was observed in the scores of emotional intelligence of control group (t= 0.683 df =18 P= 0.503) who was not imparted life skill training. The findings showed that the mean scores of emotional intelligence increased in the case group after training in life skills and the difference was significant. By performing programs such as life skill training, the level of emotional intelligence of the students could be increased which itself could lead to academic success, reduced substance abuse and increased stress tolerance among the students. Thus, it can be concluded that emotional intelligence has a major role in mental health and life skill training and could be viewed as a bridge relating emotional intelligence to mental health.

Dhanda and Singh (2014) conducted a longitudinal study to explore the influence of soft life skills of school children in rural areas of Hisar, Haryana in India. A sample of 50 children was selected with the aim to investigate the influence of fluid intelligence on soft life skills in four domains i.e. Communication Skills, Daily living Skills, Social Skills and Motor Skills. Data was collected on same children for two years. An analysis of variance for regression between these skills and fluid intelligence indicated that there was a significant as well as strong relation between these two constructs because fluid intelligence is closely related to the development of these skills.

It is revealed from the above studies that life skills training could lead to increased emotional intelligence. Considering the study results of the relationship between high emotional intelligence and mental health which reduced unhealthy behaviors, increased power of coping with the problems and academic success, it can be concluded that life skill training could lead to improved mental health and reduced unhealthy behaviors through its impact on emotional intelligence.

Life Skills and Social Adjustment

The importance of social adjustment has been seen in the behavior of adolescents in dealing with people, having control on aggressiveness and to deal with different situations. Apart from this, recent findings in behavioral epidemiology indicate that mental health problems, social problems and health risk behavior often co-occur as an organized pattern of adolescent risk behavior (Greenberg, Domitrovich, & Bumbarger, 1999). It focuses on increasing positive social skills with which to handle inevitable social disagreement and conflict, on the ability to generate alternative solutions to an interpersonal problem and on the ability to conceptualize the consequences of different behavior. Significant relationships between these problem-solving skills and social adjustment were found not only among preschool and kindergarten children but also among adolescents and adults. So, it can be said that social-cognitive skills, social competence and problem-solving skills serve as mediators for behavior, both positive and negative.

In a study on life skill education as the foundation of social maturity, Duhan (2014) investigated the impact of life skill education on social maturity skills of adolescent girls. A sample of 60 adolescent girls, aged 15 to19 years, from the rural area of Hisar, Haryana in India was selected through purposive sampling method. Results highlighted that 46.7 percent of respondents were having mature social skills followed by 36.7 percent having immature social skills before imparting intervention on life skills. Post-test results revealed a significant improvement in all aspects of social maturity skills. Results related to the mean differences in the social maturity of the respondents before and after imparting the intervention program pinpointed that the respondents differed significantly for their personal adequacy skills at pre- and post-test stage of intervention (t= 5.96). The study led to the conclusion that life skill interventions are significantly helpful to improve social adequacy skills among adolescent girls so as to enable them to deal effectively with life challenges.

Another similar study was undertaken by Pooja and Meenakshi (2014) to assess the impact of life skill education program on 100 young girls selected from Government College of Panchkula, Haryana in India in the areas of adjustment with parents, siblings, teachers and peers; self-efficacy in terms of coping with a variety of demands in life and self-esteem. Fifty girls were given life skill education for two months, comprised the experimental group and another fifty girls comprised the control group who were not given any intervention. Results of the study revealed that young girls, who were given life skill education, had better adjustment with parents, siblings, teachers and peers, better perceived self-efficacy and better self-esteem as compared to their counterparts. Results indicated that life skill education program prepared the young girls to be competent persons in a changing and competitive society. Thus, an empowered adolescent has the competence to cope with the challenges of life using the available resources in such adverse conditions.

The social, cognitive and emotional coping skills targeted by life skill programs are shown to be mediators of problem behavior and there lies the success of life skill training programs. There are research indications that teaching skills in this way, as part of broad based life skill programs, is an effective approach for primary prevention education (Errecart, Walberg, Ross,

Gold, Fiedler, & Kolbe, 1991; Caplan, Weissberg, Grober, Sivo, Grady, & Jacoby, 1992).

UNICEF Communication Initiative for Young People in Nepal

UNICEF, Nepal has created three interlinked ways to reach young people: edutainment through radio and television; communication material; and interpersonal discussions. 'Chatting with My Best Friend'is the first Nepali radio program for young people in Nepal. It is designed to interact with adolescents as another peer who speaks his/ her mind without moral judgment, to help break the silence surrounding physiological and emotional issues such as sex, love, relationships, peer pressure and conflict with parents.

'Catmandu' is the Nepal's first television program acted and directed by young people for the young people. This plot is created around the concept of life skills by putting protagonists through emotional conflicts, tough choices, setbacks and situations that demand empathy, creative and critical thinking, problem solving and other skills.

Life Skills Education Initiatives in India

A number of programs for adolescents in India have incorporated the component of life skill education. These programs have been implemented both by the government and the non-governmental organization (NGO) sector. Among the programs being implemented by the government, the most widely implemented program is Adolescence Education Programme (AEP) developed by the Ministry of Human Resource Development, Department of Education and The National AIDS Control Organization (NACO) for school going adolescent boys and girls. This program seeks to build adolescents skills in making important life decisions, improve interpersonal communication, foster egalitarian gender role attitudes and raise awareness about growing up matters as well as HIV/AIDS.

Another program named, Kishori Shakti Yojna (KSY) is being implemented in 2000 blocks covered under Integrated Child Development Services (ICDS). This program focuses on training of adolescent girls and aims at improving health, nutrition and self-development of adolescent girls in the age group of 11 to 18 years through linkages with education and life skills, thus enabling a better understanding of their environment related social issues.

SABLA- The Rajiv Gandhi Scheme for Empowerment of Adolescent Girls (RGSEAG) is a centrally sponsored program of Government of India under Ministry of Women and Child development. This program covers adolescent girls in the age group of 11 to 18 years under all Integrated Child Development Services (ICDS) projects in selected 200 districts in all states/ Union Territories. The objectives of the program are to enable the adolescent girls for self-development and empowerment, improve their health and nutrition status, promote awareness about health, hygiene, nutrition, adolescent reproductive and sexual health (ARSH) and family and child care, upgrade home-based skills and integrate with the National Skill Development Program (NSDP) for vocational skills and mainstream out of school adolescent girls into formal/ non-formal education.

- **Adolescent Health and Development Project (AHDP):** Is a project by the Rajiv Gandhi National Institute of Youth Development (RGNIYD). It has implemented life skill program that aims to promote leadership qualities and broaden the personality of young male and female adolescents the projects seek to address the imperative needs and concerns of adolescents by training on life skills, career guidance and counseling.
- **YUVA School Life Skill Programme (SLSP):** Has been initiated by Department of Education, Delhi along with SCERT. It helps to build students thinking, social and negotiating skills, learning capacities, personality, and effective relationships and promote their health.

Besides these government programs, a large number of programs have been implemented by NGO's. Notable among these are CEDPA, New Delhi, CHETNA, Ahmedabad, MAMTA, New Delhi, ICRW, New Delhi, Saksham, Deepshikha, Sankalp, Disha, Snehidhi, Swasbhiman and Yuva Mitra and so on

Despite many efforts by various government and the non- government organizations, the scenario is not very encouraging, especially for rural adolescent girls. This necessitates the need for more pragmatic and action-oriented approach. For this to happen, efforts should be directed towards incorporating life skills in the curriculum of primary education level to inculcate these healthy skills to shape and steer child's thought process in the desired direction.

More emphasis needs to be laid on all aspects of life skills, especially conflict resolution and problem solving, realizing their importance in helping youth to be equipped with better coping skills. Moreover, drug abuse and sexual abuse problems need to be tackled on a priority basis as these are taking toll on the economic productivity and morality of today's youngsters. Since more and more non- government organizations have taken the initiative by considering these life skills as a potent weapon to empower the youngsters in these challenging times, their efforts must be strengthened by governmental initiatives in such programs.

REFERENCES

American Psychiatric Association. (2000). *Diagnostic and statistical manual of mixed disorders* (4th ed.). APA.

Bandura, A. (1977). Self-Efficacy: Towards a unifying theory of behavioural change. *Psychological Review, 84*(2), 191–215. doi:10.1037/0033-295X.84.2.191 PMID:847061

Bandura, A. (1977). *Social Learning Theory*. Prentice Hall.

Bardhan, A. (2016). Life Skills Education: A Strategy for Handling Adolescents' Risk Behavior. *IOSR Journal of Humanities and Social Science, 21*(7), 92-99.

Bastian, V. A., Burns, N. R., & Nettelbeck, T. (2005). Emotional intelligence predicts life skills, but not as well as personality and cognitive abilities. *Personality and Individual Differences, 39*(6), 1135–1145. doi:10.1016/j.paid.2005.04.006

Battle, J. (1990). *Self-Esteem: The New Revolution*. Alberta, Canada: James Battle & Associates.

Behrani, P. (2011). Implementation Aspects of Life Skills Education Program in Central Board of Secondary Education Schools. *GESJ: Education Science and Psychology, 2*(19), 1512–1801.

Bhattacharya, M. S., & Sengupta, N. (2007). *Emotional Intelligence - Myth or Reality*. New Delhi: Excel Books.

Bhatti, B., Derezotes, D., Seung O. & Specht, H. (1992). Association between Child Maltreatment and Self-Esteem. In *The Social Importance of Self-Esteem*. Berkeley, CA: U.C.

Blascovich, J., & Joseph, T. (1993). Measures of Self-Esteem. In J. P. Robinson, P. R. Shaver, & L. S. Wrightsman (Eds.), *Measures of Personality and Social Psychological Attitudes* (3rd ed.; pp. 115–160). Ann Arbor, MI: Institute for Social Research.

Botvin, G.J. & Baker. (1984). *A cognitive -behavioral approach to substance abuse prevention was tested on seventh grade students from 10 sub-urban New York junior high schools*. Academic Press.

Botvin, G. J., Eng, A., & Williams, C. L. (1980). Preventing the Onset of Cigarette Smoking through Life Skills Training. *Preventive Medicine*, *9*(1), 135–143. doi:10.1016/0091-7435(80)90064-X PMID:7360727

Botvin, G. J., & Griffin, K. W. (2004). Life Skills Training: Empirical Findings and Future Directions. *The Journal of Primary Prevention*, *25*(2), 211–232. doi:10.1023/B:JOPP.0000042391.58573.5b

Botvin, G. J., Griffin, K. W., Paul, E., & Macaulay, A. P. (2003). Preventing tobacco and alcohol use among elementary school students through life skills training. *Journal of Child & Adolescent Substance Abuse*, *12*(4), 1–17. doi:10.1300/J029v12n04_01

Budhani, S. & Singh, B.B. (1996, July). Communication Support for Training Rural Youth in TRYSEM. *Indian Journal of Adult Education*, 33-37.

Caplan, M., Weissberg, R., Grober, J., Sivo, P., Grady, K., & Jacoby, C. (1992). Social Competence Promotion with Inner City and Suburban Young Adolescents: Effects on Social Adjustment and Alcohol Use. *Journal of Consulting and Clinical Psychology*, *60*(1), 56–63. doi:10.1037/0022-006X.60.1.56 PMID:1556286

Choudhary, S., Kaushik, S., & Sethi, D. (2014). *Impact of visual media regarding nutrition messages on school children*. Haryana: Developmental Prospects of Life Sills. Women Studies and Development Cell.

Corrigan, P. W., & Basit, A. (1996). Generalization of social skills training for persons with severe mental illness. *Cognitive and Behavioral Practice*, *4*(1), 191–206. doi:10.1016/S1077-7229(97)80018-1

Department of Adult and Continuing Education. (2006). *International Workshop on life skills Education for Youth Development*. University of Madras.

Dhanda, B., & Singh, C. K. (2014). *Soft Life Skill Education of Children in Relation to their Fluid Intelligence*. Haryana: Developmental Prospects of Life Sills. Women Studies and Development Cell.

Duhan, K. (2014). *Life Skill Education: The Foundation of Social Maturity*. Haryana: Developmental Prospects of Life Sills. Women Studies and Development Cell.

Duhan, K., & Aneja, A. (2014). *Life Skill for Life Time- Through Educational Programme*. Haryana: Developmental Prospects of Life Sills. Women Studies and Development Cell.

Errecart, M. T., Walberg, H. J., Ross, J. G., Gold, R. S., Fiedler, J. L., & Kolbe, L. J. (1991). Effectiveness of teenage health teaching modules. *The Journal of School Health*, *61*(1), 26–30. doi:10.1111/j.1746-1561.1991.tb07855.x PMID:2027290

Feindler, E., Ecton, R., Kingsley, D., & Dubey, D. (1986). Group anger control trainingfor institutional psychiatric male adolescents. *Behavior Therapy*, *17*(2), 109–123. doi:10.1016/S0005-7894(86)80079-X

Goleman, D. (1995). *Emotional Intelligence: Why it can matter more than IQ*. New York: Bantam Books.

Goleman, D. (1998). *Working with Emotional Intelligence*. New York: Bantam Books.

Goleman, D. (2001). An EI - based theory of performance. In C. Cherniss & D. Goleman (Eds.), *The emotionally intelligent workplace: How to select for, measure and improve emotional intelligence in individuals, groups and organizations*. San Francisco: Jossey – Bass.

Greenberg, M. T., Domitrovich, C., & Bumbarger, B. (1999). *Preventing mental disorders in school-age children: A review of the effectiveness of prevention programs*. Pennsylvania State University, Prevention Research Center for the Promotion of Human Development.

Harter, S. (1990). Identity and self-development. In S. Feldman & G. Elliott (Eds.), *At the threshold: The developing adolescent* (pp. 352–387). Cambridge, MA: Harvard University Press.

Hirsch, B., & DuBois, D. (1991). Self-esteem in early adolescence: The identification and prediction of contrasting longitudinal trajectories. *Journal of Youth and Adolescence*, *20*(1), 53–72. doi:10.1007/BF01537351 PMID:24264916

Hong, E. (1998). Different stability of individual differences in state and trait test anxiety. *Learning and Individual Differences*, *10*(1), 51–66. doi:10.1016/S1041-6080(99)80142-3

Jamali, S., Sabokdast, S., Sharif Nia, H., & Hossein, A., Goudarzian, Beik, S., & Allen, K-A. (2016). The Effect of Life Skills Training on Mental Health of Iranian Middle School Students: A Preliminary Study. *Iranian Journal of Psychiatry*, *11*(4), 269–272. PMID:28050189

Jones, B., & Iredale, N. (2006). Developing and Entrepreneurial Summer School, Innovations in Education and Teaching. *International Journal of Education*, 43–45.

Joseph, K. S. (2008). Equip yourself with life skills, Mastering life skills can elevate you to higher spheres of your private, social and professional life. The Bombay Saint Paul Society, Better Yourself Books Publishers.

Katyal, S. (2014). *Resilience: A Life Skill among Adolescents Living in Slums of Chandigarh*. Haryana: Developmental Prospects of Life Sills. Women Studies and Development Cell.

Kaur, J., & Kaur, R. (2014). *A study of Attitude of Prospective Teachers Towards Life Skill Education*. Haryana: Developmental Prospects of Life Sills. Women Studies and Development Cell.

Keefe, F. J., Caldwell, D. S., & Baucom, D. (1996). Coping skills training in the management of osteoarthritis knee pain. *Pain*, *110*(3), 539–549. doi:10.1016/j.pain.2004.03.022 PMID:15288394

Khanna, A., & Sharma, R. (2014). *Puppetry- A media for edutainment and enhancing life skills of youth*. Haryana: Developmental Prospects of Life Sills. Women Studies and Development Cell.

Khera, S., & Khosla, S. (2012). A Study Of Core Life Skills Of Adolescents In Relation To Their Self Concept Developed Through Yuva School Life Skill Programme. *International Journal of Social Science & Interdisciplinary Research, 1*(11). Retrieved from http://www.indianresearchjournals.com/pdf/ijssir/2012/november/12.pdf

Lane, J., Lane, M., & Kyprianou, A. (2004). Self-efficacy, self-esteem and their impact on Academic Performance. *Social Behavior and Personality, 32*(3), 247–256. doi:10.2224bp.2004.32.3.247

Lineo. K. (2009). Life Skills of adolescents for National development regardless of their diversity in culture, economic conditions and social and political structures. Manual for Life Skills Assessment Scale. Institute of Development Management–Lesotho. *International Journal of Social Science and Interdisciplinary Research, 1*(11).

Mangrulkar, L., Whiteman, C. V., & Posner, M. (2001). *Life Skills approach to child and adolescent healthy human development.* Washington, DC: Pan American Health Association.

Manocha, A. (2013). *Capacity building of adolescent girls through women studies and development cell.* Haryana: Developmental Prospects of Life Sills. Women Studies and Development Cell.

Matsuda, E., & Uchiyama, K. (2006). Assertion training in coping with mental disorders with psychosomatic disease. *International Congress Series, 1287*, 276–278. doi:10.1016/j.ics.2005.12.042

McCreary, M. L., Slavin, L. A., & Berry, E. J. (1996). Predicting problem behavior and self-esteem among African American Adolescents. *Journal of Adolescent Research, 11*(2), 216–234. doi:10.1177/0743554896112004

Miller, R. L. (1988). Positive self-esteem and alcohol/drug related attitudes among school children. *Journal of Alcohol and Drug Education, 33*, 26–31.

Mishara, B. L., & Ystgaard, M. (2006). Effectiveness of a mental health promotion program to improve coping skills in young children: Zippo's Friends. *Early Childhood Research Quarterly, 21*(1), 110–123. doi:10.1016/j.ecresq.2006.01.002

Nair, M.K.C. (2005). Family Life Skills and Life Skills Education for Adolescents: Trivandrum Experience. *Journal of Indian Association for Child and Adolescent Mental Health.*

Nanda, S. (2001). *Assessment of an Improved module of National Adolescent Girls Scheme and Evaluation of the Ongoing Scheme.* Unpublished doctoral dissertation, Panjab University, Chandigarh, India.

Nasser, S. G., & Soran, R. (2010). Efficacy of life skills training on increase of mental health and self-esteem of the students. *Procedia: Social and Behavioral Sciences*, (5): 1818–1822.

NCERT. (1999). Adolescents Education in Schools: Package of Basic Materials. New Delhi: NCERT.

O'Donnell, L., Stueve, A., Doval, A., Duran, R., Haber, D., Atnafou, R., ... Piessens, P. (1999). The effectiveness of the Reach for Health Community Youth Service Learning Program in reducing early and unprotected sex among urban middle school students. *American Journal of Public Health, 89*(2), 176–181. doi:10.2105/AJPH.89.2.176 PMID:9949745

Phuphaibul, R., Thanooruk, R., Leucha, Y., Sirapo-ngam, Y., & Kanobdee, C. (2005). The Impacts of the "Immune of Life" for Teens Module Application on the Coping Behaviors and Mental Health of Early Adolescents. *Journal of Pediatric Nursing, 20*(6), 461–468. doi:10.1016/j.pedn.2005.08.003 PMID:16298288

Poobalan, A. S., Pitchforth, E., Janet, M., Tucker, S., Philip, K., & Spratt, J. (2009). Characteristics of effective interventions in improving young people's sexual health: A review of reviews. *Sex Education, 9*(3), 319–336. doi:10.1080/14681810903059185

Pooja & Meenakshi. (2014). *Life Skill Education for Adjustment, Self-Efficacy and Self Esteem of Young Girls.* Haryana: Developmental Prospects of Life Sills. Women Studies and Development Cell.

Rahmati, B., Adibrad, N., Tahmasian, K., & Sedghpour, B. S. (2010). The effectiveness of life skill training on social adjustmentin children. *Procedia: Social and Behavioral Sciences, 5*, 870–874. doi:10.1016/j.sbspro.2010.07.201

Ramesht, M., & Farshad, C. (2010). *Study of life skills training in prevention of drug abuse in students.* Third seminar of students' mental health.

Rosenberg, M. (1986). *Conceiving the Self.* Krieger.

Saman, J., Sekineh, S., Hamid, S., Nia, A., Hossein, G., Sima, B., & Kelly-Ann, A. (2016). The Effect of Life Skills Training on Mental Health of Iranian Middle School Students: A Preliminary Study. *Iranian Journal of Psychiatry*, *11*(4), 269–272. PMID:28050189

Sangwan, S., Muraal, S., & Davar, V. (2014). *Strengthening knowledge towards family life education in rural women in Haryana*. Haryana: Developmental Prospects of Life Sills. Women Studies and Development Cell.

Sharma, S. (2003). Measuring life skills of adolescents in a secondary school of Kathmandu: An Experience in Kathmandu. *University Medical Journal*, *1*(3), 170-176.

Sherman, S. G., Sutcliffe, C., Srirojn, B., Latkin, C. A., Aramratanna, A., & Celentano, D. D. (2009). Evaluation of a peer network intervention trial among young methamphetamine users in Chiang Mai, Thailand. *Social Science & Medicine*, *68*(1), 69–79. doi:10.1016/j.socscimed.2008.09.061 PMID:18986746

Sikandra & Kumar, V. (2014). Impact of nutrition education on mothers of obese adolescents. Developmental Prospects of Life Sills. Women Studies and Development Cell, Haryana.

Sindhu, C. S., Rani, J., & Sangwan, S. (2014). *Nutrition Education: The Required Dimension in Life Skill Education*. Haryana: Developmental Prospects of Life Sills. Women Studies and Development Cell.

Smith, E. A. (2004). Evaluation of life Skills training and Infused-life Skills Training in a rural setting: Outcomes at two years. *Journal of Alcohol and Drug Education*.

Sukhodolsky, D. G., Golub, A., Stone, E. C., & Orban, L. (2004). Dismantling anger control training for children: A randomized pilot study of social problem-solving versus social skills training components. *Behavior Therapy*, *36*(1), 15–23. doi:10.1016/S0005-7894(05)80050-4

TACADE. (1990). Skills for the primary school children: Promoting the protection of children. Salford, UK: TACADE.

Teasdale, J. D., Segal, Z. V., Willaiams, J. M. G., Ridgeway, V. A., Soulsbuy, J. M., & Lax, M. A. (2000). Prevention of relapsed recurrence in major depression mindfulness-based Cognitive therapy. *Journal of Consulting and Clinical Psychology*, *68*(4), 615–623. doi:10.1037/0022-006X.68.4.615 PMID:10965637

Fard, J. H., Lolaty, H. A., Ghahari, S., & Tirgari, A. (2012). The Effect of Life Skills Training on Emotional Intelligence of the Medical Sciences Students in Iran. *Indian Journal of Psychological Medicine*, *34*(4), 350–354. doi:10.4103/0253-7176.108217 PMID:23723543

Trzesniewski, K. H., Donnellan, M. B., Moffitt, T. E., Robins, R. W., Poulton, R., & Caspi, A. (2006). Low self-esteem during adolescence predicts poor health, criminal behavior and limited economic prospects during adulthood. *Developmental Psychology*, *42*(2), 381–390. doi:10.1037/0012-1649.42.2.381 PMID:16569175

UNESCO. (2001). *Life Skills in Non-Formal Education: A Review*. UNESCO. Retrieved from http://www.ibe.unesco.org/fileadmin/user_upload/hiv_and_aids/publications/life_skills_in_non-formal_education.pdf

UNICEF. (2005). *Life Skills Based Education in South Asia*. Retrieved from www.Unicef.org

UNICEF. (2012). *Global Evaluation of Life Skills Programmes, Evaluation Report*. Retrieved from Error! Hyperlink reference not valid.

Vranda, M. N., & Rao, M. C. (2011). Life skills education for young adolescents–Indian experience. *Journal of the Indian Academy of Applied Psychology*, *37*(9), 9–15.

Weitlauf, J. C., Smith, R. E., & Cervon, D. (2000). Generalization Effects of Coping-Skills Training: Influence of Self-Defense Training on Women's Efficacy Beliefs, Assertiveness, and Aggression. *The Journal of Applied Psychology*, *85*(4), 625–633. doi:10.1037/0021-9010.85.4.625 PMID:10948806

Wong, C. S., Foo, M. D., Wang, C. W., & Wong, P. M. (2007). The feasibility of training and development of EI: An exploratory study in Singapore, Hong Kong and Taiwan. *Intelligence*, *35*(2), 141–150. doi:10.1016/j.intell.2006.04.008

World Health Organization. (1996). *Life Skills education for children and adolescents in schools*. Geneva: World Health Organization Programme on Mental Health.

World Health Organization. (1997). *Life Skills Education For Children And Adolescents In Schools, Introduction and Guidelines to Facilitate the Development and Implementation of Life Skills Programmes*. Geneva: WHO. Retrieved from http://www.asksource.info/pdf/31181_lifeskillsed_1994.pdf

Yadav, P., & Iqbal, N. (2009). Impact of Life Skill Training on Self-esteem, Adjustment and Empathy among Adolescents. *Journal of the Indian Academy of Applied Psychology*, *35*(10), 61–70.

Young, M., Kelley, R., & Denny, G. (1997). Evaluation of selected life skill modules from the contemporary health series with students in grade. *Perceptual and Motor Skills*, *84*(3), 811–818. doi:10.2466/pms.1997.84.3.811 PMID:9172187

Zollinger, T. W., Commings, S. F., & Caine, V. (2003). Impact of the life skills training curriculum on middle school student's tobacco use in Marion County, Indiana. *Life Skills Education: A Strategy for Handling Adolescents' Risk Behavior*. Retrieved from http://scertdelhi.nic.in/yuva.html http://socialwelfare.icdsbih.gov.in/Schemes-Programmes.php

Chapter 6
Summary and Conclusion

ABSTRACT

Adolescence is the transitional phase, which is formative, impressionable, and hence, vulnerable. The healthy development of adolescents depends on several interactive and complex factors like socio-economic and environmental factors in which they are born and brought up, the interpersonal relationships they develop with peers and adults, values of the community, and the available opportunities for education and employment. For the health management of adolescents, "psychological and interpersonal skills" need to be acquired to help them to communicate better, to make more informed and balanced decisions, to avoid risky situations, and to cope with stress as these life skills shape attitudes and ultimately lead to pro-social behavior and productive lifestyles. Moreover, the importance of designing health services that can attract and engage adolescents, create opportunities to discuss sensitive health and behavioral issues, and offer high-quality care as well as guidance for health promotion and disease prevention cannot be undermined.

KEY FACTS

- Adolescents represent one fifth of the global population; healthy and competent adolescents who enter the workforce can raise the economic productivity of a country.
- Investing in the health of adolescents, in general, can help prevent the estimated 1.4 million deaths that occur globally every year because of road traffic injuries, violence, suicide, HIV and pregnancy-related causes in this age group.

DOI: 10.4018/978-1-5225-7384-5.ch006

- It can also improve the health and well-being of many millions of adolescents who experience health problems such as depression or anemia.
- Economists stress the importance of using this "demographic dividend" to reap the benefits of having a growing cohort of working age adults relative to the dependent population for national development. (United Nations Population Fund, 2013)

INTRODUCTION

According to the World Health Organization (1995), "One of the most important commitments a country can make for future economic, social and political progress and stability is to address the health and development needs of its adolescents." Adolescence is a time of major transition between childhood and adulthood. It is a period when significant physical, psychological and behavioral changes occur and when young people develop many of the habits, behaviors and relationships they will carry into their adult lives. The health system has a crucial role to play in promoting healthful behavior and preventing disease during adolescence.

The health of adolescents can be defined by traditional measures (mortality rates, incidence of disease and the prevalence of chronic conditions). A more complex and complete picture of adolescent health status, however, also encompasses the prevalence of various leading adolescent behaviors and health outcomes as well as health indicators that may adversely affect their health status in adulthood.

The period between 10-19 years of age is the period when one is young and still in a growing stage in an individual's life. This is a period when the individual experiences a growth spurt in all areas of development i.e., physical, cognitive, social and emotional. Those in the age of 16-18 years are almost like adults. The period is definitely marked by rapid physical growth in the body and also change in body shape. The most noticeable changes in boys are broad shoulders, oily skin, facial hair, muscular body and cracked or deep voice. Similarly, girls have narrow waistline and wide hips, oily skin, enlarged breasts and shrill voice. Almost 25 percent of adult height and about 50 percent of adult weight are gained during this period. Thus, the importance of adequate nutrition and exercise, healthy and hygienic habits at this stage are important and obvious.

Growth is also occurring at a very rapid pace in the reproductive organs and release of hormones that is not properly regulated initially leading to mood swings. The beginning of the menstrual cycle in girls and wet dreams in boys can be all very frightening if correct and timely information is not provided to them. Lack of information or misinformation regarding these leads to many doubts, fears, confusion and worries. Myths and misconceptions abound among the adolescents.

On the emotional front, adolescents get anxious and imagine physical faults in their body structure and shape. This is mainly because they are preoccupied all the time with their body image. They spend a lot of time in making it acceptable to themselves. There is a strong attraction towards the opposite sex during this period. Rebellious thoughts; desire to break away from accepted social norms and the family, moods ranging from elation to depression, etc. are some of the other common emotions experienced by them. They need to be told repeatedly that all this is a normal part of growing up because adolescents find it difficult to understand and accept these changes. Somehow, they find solace in the company of peers. They feel that their peers are the only ones who can understand them and their problems.

Socially, since peer group becomes very important, they like to spend a lot of time together and like to do things which everybody else is doing. This may result in positive or negative influences. If positive, they develop spirit of competition, cooperation, achievement, empathy, etc. They have a great desire to help each other and be fair to each other. Adolescents generally want to be in the company of their age-mates because they feel that they are better understood there. This is also an expression to their desire to break away from adults and establish an identity of their own. Although, this is a natural outcome of the process of growing up, adolescents often have to face adult wrath for such actions and consequently, they grow tense and rebel.

This is an age which is formative, impressionable and therefore most vulnerable. The social environment during this period plays a very important role in influencing the adolescents. It is a phase of opportunities as well as risks making and it very easy for a young person to get influenced, positively or negatively. Learning to make informed choices, keep off infections like HIV/AIDS and addictions to drugs, alcohol, etc., and adopt a responsible behaviour leading to a healthy individual is most important at this stage.

Cognitively, they have reached a stage when they can do abstract thinking and understand other people's perspective. They love speculating for best alternative and do problem solving. They can now solve problems by making assumptions, analyzing, connecting or disconnecting, relating, etc. They can identify the uncontrollable factors and understand the need to take precautions.

Preparation for a vocation/ profession is an important goal before them and they do tend to put in the needed efforts. Career counseling can, not only guide them to choose the right avenue and direct their energies to right channels, but also help them to ease out their tensions.

As a child moves through the school years into adolescence, prevention of behavior that can lead to health risks takes a great importance. Many habits and lifestyle choices that start during these critical years contribute greatly to the overall health of the adults. WHO estimates that nearly 70 percent of premature deaths among adults are largely due to behavior initiated during adolescence. Thus, major health issues of adolescents are related to physical and reproductive health and emotional maturity so as to have sound mental health.

The 12 million girls born every year in India, who have been most vulnerable for centuries and are even today, vulnerable to the insults of poverty and deprivation, form the foundation. Studies have shown that of the 12 million girls born in India every year, 1.5 million girls die before the age of one and one out of every four does not live to celebrate her fifteenth birthday. In spite of having a biological advantage over boys, 0.3 million more girls than boys die with an estimated one in every six female deaths due to gender discrimination and gross neglect. This can be linked to neglect of females as infants, as children, as adolescents and as mothers.

Accidents, violence and suicides are the three most common causes of death among adolescents. Impaired mental and emotional health is a precursor or consequence of many health-risk behaviors, such as alcohol and substance abuse; unwanted or unprotected sex; physical, sexual or emotional abuse; reckless driving or excessive risk taking; extreme eating habits and excessive influence of advertisement or other forms of media. Other behavior and attitudes are also integrally linked to adolescent mental health. These dilemmas arise out of everyday issues like peer influence, dating identity, emerging sexuality, independence, separation, identity crises, anxiety and responsibility as well as more serious ones like violent behavior, experimental sex, teen suicides and other disorders. The impact of all these negative influences can be very damaging and hence needs proper and timely intervention.

Of the population affected by AIDS/HIV, over 35 percent belong to the 15-25-year age group. Similarly, 24 percent of drug abusers are in the age group of 12 to 18 years. Most of the people who pick up the habit of smoking or drinking alcohol also do so in their adolescence and more often than not, the reason for beginning these behaviours is the effect of peer pressure.

This is also an age of risk taking and experimentation. In the company of peers, they try out things which can land them into trouble. Saying no to such actions is difficult and a reason to be tense. More so, because they are learning to build relationships with people outside their homes and at no cost they want to spoil these relationships. What they need is to build up are their negotiation skills and use these to understand the physical and emotional boundaries within relationships and say 'NO', wherever and whenever needed. They also need to learn to influence people to get them involved in constructive and positive behaviors.

An important reason for feeling tense at this stage is no set goal for future vocation/ profession. Consequently, they find it difficult to concentrate on studies; begin to experience examination stress and career related anxiety. Adolescents are worried about their future, about their bodies, about the physical growth that has taken place, about their intellect, about their social relationship with peers and adults, about gender discrimination, about any bad company they have contacted and bad habits they may have picked up etc. They may have already formed some opinions about certain things and may be in the process of forming opinions about certain other things. They are under lot of pressure from their peers about many things, including experimentation and defying parents and adults. In short, they are on the lookout for help, assurance and clarifications.

The emotional maturity level of each adolescent is different and so is their reaction to each situation. Physical appearance is a particularly important psychological construct associated with social acceptance among adolescents. In order for adolescents to take the risks that are important for their development and avoid those that will do them an irreparable harm, their right to health and development needs to be fulfilled. This includes their right to information and acquisition of skills, a range of health care services, a safe and supportive environment and opportunities to participate.

'Life skills' are the abilities for adaptive and positive behavior that enables individual to deal effectively with the demands and challenges of everyday life (WHO, 2003). UNICEF uses the term to describe 'psychological and interpersonal skills' which help people to communicate better, to make more informed and balanced decisions, to avoid risky situations, or to cope with stress. It is believed that along with the necessary knowledge, these skills are considered important because they can shape attitudes and ultimately lead to pro-social behavior and productive life styles.

For an adolescent, learning life skills is important because life skills are a group of psychosocial competencies and interpersonal skills which help them to make informed decisions, communicate effectively and develop coping and self-management skills to lead a healthy and productive life.

Researches indicate that life skills help a person to understand himself, his friends and the world around. By sharing positive life skill lessons, the learner becomes more effective and discovers his strengths and weaknesses and interests in life. It is also revealed that these skills are learnt by observing, practicing and by application. This can best happen at home under the guidance of parents and in school under the supervision or friendly guidance.

Life skill approach is an interactive process of teaching and learning, which focuses equally on acquiring knowledge, attitudes and skills. It strengthens educational process by insisting on participatory and gender sensitive teaching and learning methods. Such methods allow all participants (including facilitator) equal opportunities to listen to and learn from each other. It is a good interactive educational methodology which focuses not on just giving information but also on bringing about a change in behavior and attitude of the adolescents.

The life skill approach includes interpersonal and psychosocial skills e.g., assertion, negotiation, decision-making, empathy building, value clarification, and coping skills. This is an important component of the whole process because for bringing a change in behavior, mere information is not enough. In other words, the approach is designed for learning and not teaching how to bring change in behaviour. The methods used in inculcating life skills are simple and based on experiential learning (learning by doing). The approach has been extensively tried for imparting health related messages to adolescents but can be equally effective in imparting knowledge in any other subject area.

The most important characteristics of instructional design suited for learning life skills are interaction and experience. Multiple teaching- learning styles like discussions, investigation, working in small group, problem solving, peer tutoring/ cooperative learning, project work, etc., are suggested methodologies because these involve the interaction and the opportunities for experiential learning. All these methods are no different from the ones used while helping the learners in contact program. The only difference is that for developing life skills one chooses situations that are closer to life so that these enable the learner to have a feel of the content to be learned.

The key recommendations are to link the provision of sexuality education and sexual and reproductive health (SRH) services; build awareness, acceptance, and support for youth-friendly SRH education and services; address gender inequality in terms of beliefs, attitudes, and norms; and target the early adolescent period (10-14 years). The many knowledge gaps, however, point to the pressing need for further research on how to best design effective adolescent SRH intervention packages and how best to deliver them.

There is strong public health, human rights, and economic reasons to invest in adolescent's health. Promoting mutually respectful attitudes between and among adolescent girls and boys in connection with sexuality as well as other healthy behaviors (e.g., reducing the harmful use of alcohol and other substances) will form the foundation for the good health of populations as adolescents become adults and for social and economic development more broadly. Investing in the health of adolescents in general can help prevent the estimated 1.4 million deaths that occur globally every year because of road traffic injuries, violence, suicide, HIV, and pregnancy-related causes in this age group. It can also improve the health and well-being of many millions of adolescents who experience health problems such as depression or anemia (State of the World Population, 2013).

There is also growing recognition of the economic benefits of investing in the healthy development of adolescents and the economic costs of not doing so. Adolescents represent one fifth of the global population; healthy competent adolescents who enter the workforce can raise the economic productivity of a country. Economists stress the importance of using this "demographic dividend" to reap the benefits of having a growing cohort of working age adults relative to the dependent population for national development. However, this requires an investment in human and physical capital that enables adolescents and young people to stay healthy, get educated, and find productive and income-generating employment (Mohajer & Earnest, 2010; UNPF, 2010).

Researches from various sources and the experiences of adolescents and health care providers, health organizations and research centers suggest the importance of designing health services that can attract and engage adolescents, create opportunities to discuss sensitive health and behavioral issues and offer high-quality care as well as guidance for health promotion and disease prevention. Consistent with these findings and views, a variety of national and international organizations have defined critical elements of health systems that would improve adolescents' access to appropriate services, highlighted design elements that would improve the quality of those services, and identified ways to foster patient–provider relationships that can lead to better health for adolescents.

World Health Organization (1995) has identified five characteristics that constitute objectives for responsive adolescent health services:

- **Accessible:** Policies and procedures ensure that services are broadly accessible.
- **Acceptable:** Policies and procedures consider culture and relationships and the climate of engagement.
- **Appropriate:** Health services fulfill the needs of all young people.
- **Effective:** Health services reflect evidence-based standards of care and professional guidelines.
- **Equitable:** Policies and procedures do not restrict the provision of and eligibility for services.

These five objectives provide a valuable framework for assessing the use, adequacy, and quality of adolescent health services; comparing the extent to which different services, settings and providers meet the health needs of young people; identifying the gaps that keep services from achieving these objectives and recommending ways to close these gaps.

However, many adolescent health services and settings take a limited, problem-oriented approach and focus on care for certain health conditions or specific issues, thus failing to meet the broader needs and behavioral challenges that characterizes adolescence. Because of this narrow focus, many providers of health services are poorly equipped to foster disease prevention and health promotion for adolescents. This is especially true in the areas of mental health, oral health and substance abuse as well as services that address sexual behavior and reproductive health.

Many medical professionals recognize the importance of parents' involvement in their decisions regarding adolescent's health care. At the same time, however, privacy concerns influence adolescents' willingness to seek services at all, their choice of provider, their candor in giving a health history, their willingness to accept specific services and other important aspects of access to care. A balance is needed between maintaining the confidentiality of information and records regarding care for which adolescent minors are allowed to give their consent and encouraging the involvement of parents and families in the health care services received by adolescents whenever possible, both supporting and respecting their role and importance in adolescents' lives and health care.

Moreover, regulatory bodies would need to involve specialists and educators/scholars within relevant disciplines to define competencies in adolescent health. They would also have to require professionals who serve adolescents in health care settings to complete a minimum amount of education in basic areas of adolescent development, health issues unique to this life stage and a life skill framework that encourages providers to focus on helping the adolescent develop healthful habits that can be carried forward into their adult lives.

Finally, agencies that fund training programs would have to adhere to the requirements of the regulatory bodies (i.e., with regard to accreditation, licensure and certification, and to maintenance of licensure or certification where appropriate) and content on adolescent health care would have to be mandatory in all relevant training programs.

To conclude, it can be said that healthy development of adolescents depends on several interactive and complex factors like socio-economic and environmental factors in which they are born and brought up, the interpersonal relationships they develop with their peers and other adults around them, values of the community in which they live and the opportunities they have for education and employment. If there are pressures and stresses due to expectations from adults and peers, conflicts with siblings, peers and adults, due to relationships with same and opposite sex members of the family, friends and community and due to competition arising in education and job market, they need to learn to cope up with these pressures. Such issues are seldom addressed either in the family or elsewhere. Neither does it is realized that appreciation, if they are doing a good job of coping and counseling and guidance if they are not, enhances their self-esteem and helps them in making good adjustments in life. A timely help in any form can go a long way in establishing them in their endeavor.

REFERENCES

Bhagbanprakash. (2000). *21st Century: Development Challenges*. Commonwealth Youth Programme Asia Centre, Commonwealth Secretariat, Asia Centre, Chandigarh.

DPED. (1995). *Empowering the Girl Child Through Education-DPED Strategies to Address Gender Disparities*. Educational Consultants India Limited.

Learner's Guide for out of School Adolescents. (2002). Population and Development, United Agency Working Group.

Mohajer, N., & Earnest, J. (2010). Widening the aim of health promotion to include the most disadvantaged: Vulnerable adolescents and the social determinants of health. *Health Education Research*, *25*(3), 387–394. doi:10.1093/her/cyq016 PMID:20332180

Puri, N. (1998). The girl child in India. *The Journal of Family Welfare*, *44*(3), 1–8.

Tanner, J. M. (1990). *Foetus into man: physical growth from conception to maturity*. Cambridge, MA: Harvard University Press.

UNESCO. (n.d.). Retrieved from www.unesco.org/education

UNICEF. (n.d.a). *Life Skills – Quality Education*. Retrieved from www.unicef.org/lifeskills

UNICEF. (n.d.b). *Teacher Talking*. Retrieved from www.unicef.org/education

United Nations Population Fund. (2010). *The case for investing in young people*. New York: United Nations Population Fund.

United Nations Population Fund. (2013). *State of the World Population Motherhood in childhood: Facing the challenge in adolescent pregnancy*. United Nations. Retrieved from http://www.peacecorps.gov/library/pdf/M0063_lifeskillscomplete.pdf

WFS. (1995). *Too old for toys- Too young for babies: Glimpses of Childhood in India*. WFS.

World Health Organization. (1995). *United Nations Population Fund, and United Nations Children's Fund Action for Adolescent Health: Towards a Common Agenda: Recommendations from a Joint Study Group*. Available: http://www.who.int/child_adolescent_health/documents/frh_adh_97_9/en/index.html

World Health Organization. (2003). *Module on Adolescent Mental Health: Programme on Adolescent Mental Health, Health and Behaviour Unit*. New Delhi: Department of Sustainable Development and Healthy Environment, WHO Regional Office for South East Asia.

Glossary

ACC/SCN: Administrative Committee on Co-Ordination/Sub-Committee on Nutrition.

ADHD: Attention deficit hyperactivity disorder.

AEP: Adolescence education programme.

AHDP: Adolescent Health and Development Project.

AISS: Adjustment inventory for school students.

ANCOVA: Analysis of Co-variance.

ANOVA: Analysis of variance.

ARSH: Adolescent reproductive and sexual health.

ASRHR: Adolescent sexual and reproductive health and rights.

AYA: Adolescents and young adults.

BDI: Beck's depression inventory.

BMI: Body mass index.

BMIZ: Z scores of body mass index for age.

BSS: Beck scale for suicide ideation.

C-GAS: Children's global assessment scale.

CBEP: Classroom-based educational programs.

CBM: Cognitive behaviour modification.

CBPT: Cognitive behavioural play therapy.

CBSE: Central Board of Secondary Education.

CBT: Cognitive behaviour therapy.

CCE: Continuous and comprehensive evaluation.

CDC: Centers for Disease Control and Prevention.

CED: Chronic energy deficiency.

CEDAW: Convention on the Elimination of Discrimination Against Women.

CMHAP: Comprehensive mental health action plan.

CPMS: Childhood psychopathology measurement schedule.

CRC: Committee on Rights of the Child.

CSE: Comprehensive sexuality education.

DALYs: Disability-adjusted life years.

DASS: Depression anxiety stress scale.

DAWBA: Development and wellbeing assessment.

DISC-C: Diagnostic interview schedule for children-parent informant.

DISC-P: Diagnostic interview schedule for children-child informant.

DSM-IV: Diagnostic and Statistical Manual-IV.

EFA: Education for all.

EQ: Empathy quotient.

FGM/C: Female genital mutilation/cutting.

FSH: Follicle stimulating hormone.

FSW: Female sex worker.

FTN: Felt treatment needs.

G-6-PD: Glucose 6 phosphate dehydrogenase.

GAA-HA: Global accelerated action for the health of adolescents.

GAOWG: General Assembly's Open Working Group.

GHQ-12: Twelve-item general health questionnaire.

GSWCAH: Global strategy for women's, children's, and adolescents' health.

GYTS: Global youth tobacco surveys.

HAZ: Z scores of height for age.

HIV/AIDS: Human immuno-deficiency virus.

IAP: Indian Association of Paediatrics.

ICD: International classification of diseases.

ICDS: Integrated child development services.

ICMR: Indian Council of Medical Research.

ICPD: International Conference on Population and Development.

IDA: Iron deficiency anaemia.

IDD: Iodine deficiency disorder.

IHDC: International health and development community.

IIPS: International Institute for Population Sciences.

IOTF: International Obesity Task Force.

IPT: Inter-personal therapy.

IRDP: Integrated rural development program.

KAB: Knowledge, attitudes, and behavior.

KAP: Knowledge, attitudes, and practices.

KSY: Kishori Shakti Yojna.

LMICs: Low middle income countries.

LRTIs: Lower respiratory tract infections.

LSP: Life skill programme.

LST: Life skill training.

MANOVA: Multivariate analysis of variance.

MCH: Maternal and child health.

MCH: Mean cell haemoglobin.

MCHC: Mean cell haemoglobin concentration.

MCV: Mean cell volume.

MDG: Millennium Development Goals.

MHFW: Ministry of Health and Family Welfare.

mhGAP: Mental health gap action programme.

MHRD: Ministry of Human Resource Development.

MUAC: Mid upper arm circumference.

MYTRI: Mobilizing youth for tobacco-related initiatives in India.

NACO: National AIDS Control Organization.

NCDs: Non-communicable diseases.

NCERT: National Council of Educational Research and Training.

NCHS: National Centre for Health Statistics.

NFE: Non-formal education.

NFHS: National family health survey.

NFI: Nutrition Foundation of India.

NGO: Non-government organisation.

NHHCC: Nutrition, health, hygiene, and child care.

NHS: National Household Survey.

NIMHANS: National Institute of Mental Health and Neuro-Sciences.

NIN: National Institute of Nutrition.

NNMB: National Nutrition Monitoring Bureau.

NPU: Net protein utilization.

NRC: National Research Council.

ODL: Open and distance learning.

PAL: Physical activity level.

PEM: Protein energy malnutrition.

PIS: Parent interview schedule.

PoA: Program of action.

PPS: Proportionate probability sampling.

PVTG: Particularly vulnerable tribal group.

RDA: Recommended dietary allowances.

REPT: Rational emotive behaviour therapy.

RGNIYD: Rajiv Gandhi National Institute of Youth Development.

RGSEAG: Rajiv Gandhi Scheme for Empowerment of Adolescent Girls.

RHIME: Representative, re-sampled, routine household interview of mortality with medical evaluation.

RTIs: Road traffic injuries.

SDG: Sustainable development goal.

SDQ: Strengths and difficulties questionnaire.

SEAR: South East Asian Region.

SES: Socio-economic status.

SIT: Stress inoculation training.

SLD: Specific learning disability.

SLP: School life skill programme.

SRE: Sex and relationship education.

SRH: Sexual and reproductive health.

SRHS: Sexual and reproductive health services.

SSA: Sub-Saharan Africa.

STAI: State-trait anxiety inventory.

STI: Sexually transmitted infections.

TACADE: Teachers Advisory Committee on Alcohol and Drug Education.

TIBC: Total iron binding capacity.

TRYSEM: Training rural youth for self-employment.

UAE: United Arab Emirates.

UK: United Kingdom.

UN: United Nations.

UNESCO: United Nations Education Scientific and Cultural Organisation.

UNICEF: United Nations Children's Fund.

UNODC: United Nations Office on Drugs and Crime.

WAZ: Z scores of weight for age.

WFS: Women's feature service.

WHO: World Health Organization.

WHS: World health survey.

WYR: World youth report.

Y-PSC: Youth report of paediatric symptom checklist.

YUVA: Youth for unity and voluntary action.

Related Readings

To continue IGI Global's long-standing tradition of advancing innovation through emerging research, please find below a compiled list of recommended IGI Global book chapters and journal articles in the areas of mental health, emotional growth, and adolescent and student health. These related readings will provide additional information and guidance to further enrich your knowledge and assist you with your own research.

Al Ja'am, J. M., Abou El-Seoud, M. S., Dandashi, A., & Karkar, A. (2016). A Cognitive and Augmentative Communication System for Special Needs Education. In M. Gordon (Ed.), *Challenges Surrounding the Education of Children with Chronic Diseases* (pp. 323–342). Hershey, PA: IGI Global. doi:10.4018/978-1-4666-9452-1.ch015

Amos, Y. T. (2016). Guest Students: Faculty Expectations of Japanese International Students. In K. Bista & C. Foster (Eds.), *Exploring the Social and Academic Experiences of International Students in Higher Education Institutions* (pp. 260–291). Hershey, PA: IGI Global. doi:10.4018/978-1-4666-9749-2.ch014

Arden, M., Manathunga, C., & Bottrell, D. (2017). Internationalisation and Identity: Identity Construction Through Australian University Student Mobility Program. In A. Shahriar & G. Syed (Eds.), *Student Culture and Identity in Higher Education* (pp. 1–17). Hershey, PA: IGI Global. doi:10.4018/978-1-5225-2551-6.ch001

Athota, V. S. (2017). Foundations and Future of Well-Being: How Personality Influences Happiness and Well-Being. In S. Háša & R. Brunet-Thornton (Eds.), *Impact of Organizational Trauma on Workplace Behavior and Performance* (pp. 279–294). Hershey, PA: IGI Global. doi:10.4018/978-1-5225-2021-4.ch012

B. N. R., Prasad, B. V., & Tavaragi, M. S. (2017). Legal Aspects of Chronic Mental Illness. In B. Prasad (Ed.), Chronic Mental Illness and the Changing Scope of Intervention Strategies, Diagnosis, and Treatment (pp. 225-235). Hershey, PA: IGI Global. doi:10.4018/978-1-5225-0519-8.ch012

Bang, L. (2015). Mapping [Capital v.2.0]: An Encounter of Thoughts. In T. Hansson (Ed.), Contemporary Approaches to Activity Theory: Interdisciplinary Perspectives on Human Behavior (pp. 337-352). Hershey, PA: IGI Global. doi:10.4018/978-1-4666-6603-0.ch020

Banks, S. (2017). Mirrors of Opportunity: Joint Project of Japanese and International Students. In A. Shahriar & G. Syed (Eds.), *Student Culture and Identity in Higher Education* (pp. 18–37). Hershey, PA: IGI Global. doi:10.4018/978-1-5225-2551-6.ch002

Bedi, D. (2017). Efficacy of Art Therapy in Treating Patients with Paranoid Schizophrenia. In B. Prasad (Ed.), *Chronic Mental Illness and the Changing Scope of Intervention Strategies, Diagnosis, and Treatment* (pp. 308–320). Hershey, PA: IGI Global. doi:10.4018/978-1-5225-0519-8.ch017

Behrani, P., & Deka, D. B. (2016). Concerns for Individuals with Intellectual Disability in India. In R. Gopalan (Ed.), *Handbook of Research on Diagnosing, Treating, and Managing Intellectual Disabilities* (pp. 204–219). Hershey, PA: IGI Global. doi:10.4018/978-1-5225-0089-6.ch011

Bhargava, S., & Umrigar, D. M. (2016). Intellectual Disability in the Family Context: Parents with Intellectual Disability. In R. Gopalan (Ed.), *Handbook of Research on Diagnosing, Treating, and Managing Intellectual Disabilities* (pp. 370–385). Hershey, PA: IGI Global. doi:10.4018/978-1-5225-0089-6.ch019

Billington, R. (2017). A Critique on the Factors that Influence Mental Health Workforce Training in Developing Countries. In M. Smith & A. Jury (Eds.), *Workforce Development Theory and Practice in the Mental Health Sector* (pp. 130–143). Hershey, PA: IGI Global. doi:10.4018/978-1-5225-1874-7.ch006

Bingham, H. M. (2017). Undergraduate Nursing Curriculum Content Focuses on Emerging Issues that Influence Health. In M. Smith & A. Jury (Eds.), *Workforce Development Theory and Practice in the Mental Health Sector* (pp. 182–199). Hershey, PA: IGI Global. doi:10.4018/978-1-5225-1874-7.ch009

Bordoloi, S. D. (2016). Addressing the Needs of F-2 Wives in the United States: A Comparison of Two Educational Institutions. In K. Bista & C. Foster (Eds.), *Exploring the Social and Academic Experiences of International Students in Higher Education Institutions* (pp. 115–131). Hershey, PA: IGI Global. doi:10.4018/978-1-4666-9749-2.ch007

Bunda, T., Qi, J., Manathunga, C., & Singh, M. J. (2017). Enhancing the Australian Doctoral Experience: Locating Culture and Identity at the Centre. In A. Shahriar & G. Syed (Eds.), *Student Culture and Identity in Higher Education* (pp. 143–159). Hershey, PA: IGI Global. doi:10.4018/978-1-5225-2551-6.ch009

Byrd-Poller, L., Farmer, J. L., & Ford, V. (2017). The Role of Leaders in Facilitating Healing After Organizational Trauma. In S. Háša & R. Brunet-Thornton (Eds.), *Impact of Organizational Trauma on Workplace Behavior and Performance* (pp. 318–340). Hershey, PA: IGI Global. doi:10.4018/978-1-5225-2021-4.ch014

Cejka, P., & Mohelska, H. (2017). National Culture Influence on Organisational Trauma: A Conceptual Framework Review. In S. Háša & R. Brunet-Thornton (Eds.), *Impact of Organizational Trauma on Workplace Behavior and Performance* (pp. 162–186). Hershey, PA: IGI Global. doi:10.4018/978-1-5225-2021-4.ch007

Chen, B., & Luppicini, R. (2017). The New Era of Bullying: A Phenomenological Study of University Students' Past Experience with Cyberbullying. *International Journal of Cyber Behavior, Psychology and Learning*, *7*(2), 72–90. doi:10.4018/IJCBPL.2017040106

Chowhan, S., & Patowary, P. (2016). Issues and Recent Trends in the Assessment and Management of ID in Childhood. In R. Gopalan (Ed.), *Handbook of Research on Diagnosing, Treating, and Managing Intellectual Disabilities* (pp. 186–203). Hershey, PA: IGI Global. doi:10.4018/978-1-5225-0089-6.ch010

Cleve, R. A., Işık, İ., & Pecanha, V. D. (2017). Sexual Identities in the Workplace: Avoiding Organizational Trauma When Disclosure Occurs – Current Perspectives. In S. Háša & R. Brunet-Thornton (Eds.), *Impact of Organizational Trauma on Workplace Behavior and Performance* (pp. 188–220). Hershey, PA: IGI Global. doi:10.4018/978-1-5225-2021-4.ch008

Cook, B. L. (2016). Effectively Teaching Stressed Students. In K. Pandey & P. Upadhyay (Eds.), *Promoting Global Peace and Civic Engagement through Education* (pp. 228–241). Hershey, PA: IGI Global. doi:10.4018/978-1-5225-0078-0.ch013

Coombs, T., Burgess, P., Dickson, R., & McKay, R. (2017). Routine Outcome Measurement and the Development of the Australian Mental Health Workforce: The First 25 Years of Implementation Are the Hardest. In M. Smith & A. Jury (Eds.), *Workforce Development Theory and Practice in the Mental Health Sector* (pp. 302–316). Hershey, PA: IGI Global. doi:10.4018/978-1-5225-1874-7.ch015

Dang, C. T., & Kline, S. L. (2015). "I Can't Afford for You to Flunk": Positive Asian Stereotypes and Supportive Communication for Asian College Students. In N. Hartlep (Ed.), *Modern Societal Impacts of the Model Minority Stereotype* (pp. 1–34). Hershey, PA: IGI Global. doi:10.4018/978-1-4666-7467-7.ch001

de Soir, E., & Kleber, R. (2017). Understanding the Core of Psychological Trauma: Trauma in Contemporary French Theory. In S. Háša & R. Brunet-Thornton (Eds.), *Impact of Organizational Trauma on Workplace Behavior and Performance* (pp. 57–75). Hershey, PA: IGI Global. doi:10.4018/978-1-5225-2021-4.ch003

Dehuri, B. K., & Mukund, B. (2016). Recent Trends and Issues in Vocational Rehabilitation of People with ID. In R. Gopalan (Ed.), *Handbook of Research on Diagnosing, Treating, and Managing Intellectual Disabilities* (pp. 283–309). Hershey, PA: IGI Global. doi:10.4018/978-1-5225-0089-6.ch015

Dixon, K. V., Gonzalez-Carriedo, R., & Dixon-Krauss, L. (2017). The Implementation and Analysis of an International Student Teaching Program. In L. Leavitt, S. Wisdom, & K. Leavitt (Eds.), *Cultural Awareness and Competency Development in Higher Education* (pp. 168–188). Hershey, PA: IGI Global. doi:10.4018/978-1-5225-2145-7.ch010

Dorado, D. A., & Fass-Holmes, B. (2016). Academic Achievement and Demographics of International Undergraduates. In K. Bista & C. Foster (Eds.), *Exploring the Social and Academic Experiences of International Students in Higher Education Institutions* (pp. 233–259). Hershey, PA: IGI Global. doi:10.4018/978-1-4666-9749-2.ch013

Eapen, V., & Walter, A. (2016). Mind the Gap: Developmental Vulnerability and Mental Health. In R. Gopalan (Ed.), *Handbook of Research on Diagnosing, Treating, and Managing Intellectual Disabilities* (pp. 11–32). Hershey, PA: IGI Global. doi:10.4018/978-1-5225-0089-6.ch002

Enerstvedt, R. T. (2015). Reflections on the Theory of Activity. In T. Hansson (Ed.), *Contemporary Approaches to Activity Theory: Interdisciplinary Perspectives on Human Behavior* (pp. 353–363). Hershey, PA: IGI Global. doi:10.4018/978-1-4666-6603-0.ch021

Eriksson, I. (2015). Constitution of Objects in DWR Activity. In T. Hansson (Ed.), *Contemporary Approaches to Activity Theory: Interdisciplinary Perspectives on Human Behavior* (pp. 304–321). Hershey, PA: IGI Global. doi:10.4018/978-1-4666-6603-0.ch018

Farrell, H. J. (2016). Imagining Social Equity. In M. Gordon (Ed.), *Challenges Surrounding the Education of Children with Chronic Diseases* (pp. 247–261). Hershey, PA: IGI Global. doi:10.4018/978-1-4666-9452-1.ch012

Fellus, O. O., & Fellus, D. P. (2016). Living with ADHD: Timing Perceptions and Their Applicability to the Experience of ADHD. In M. Gordon (Ed.), *Challenges Surrounding the Education of Children with Chronic Diseases* (pp. 117–136). Hershey, PA: IGI Global. doi:10.4018/978-1-4666-9452-1.ch006

Fellus, Y. M., & Fellus, I. A. (2016). The Experience of Cancer and Asthma in the Pediatric Patient: A Family Physician's Perspective. In M. Gordon (Ed.), *Challenges Surrounding the Education of Children with Chronic Diseases* (pp. 12–25). Hershey, PA: IGI Global. doi:10.4018/978-1-4666-9452-1.ch002

Ferholt, B., Nilsson, M., Jansson, A., & Alnervik, K. (2015). Creativity in Education: Play and Exploratory Learning. In T. Hansson (Ed.), *Contemporary Approaches to Activity Theory: Interdisciplinary Perspectives on Human Behavior* (pp. 264–284). Hershey, PA: IGI Global. doi:10.4018/978-1-4666-6603-0.ch016

Firdaus, J., & Jadeja, M. (2016). Quality of Life of People with Intellectual Disability. In R. Gopalan (Ed.), *Handbook of Research on Diagnosing, Treating, and Managing Intellectual Disabilities* (pp. 139–155). Hershey, PA: IGI Global. doi:10.4018/978-1-5225-0089-6.ch008

G., L. (2017). Psychosocial Intervention Studies for Street Children with Substance Abuse. In B. Prasad (Ed.), *Chronic Mental Illness and the Changing Scope of Intervention Strategies, Diagnosis, and Treatment* (pp. 237-257). Hershey, PA: IGI Global. doi:10.4018/978-1-5225-0519-8.ch013

Gallego, J. (2017). Organizational Trauma and Change Management. In S. Háša & R. Brunet-Thornton (Eds.), *Impact of Organizational Trauma on Workplace Behavior and Performance* (pp. 140–161). Hershey, PA: IGI Global. doi:10.4018/978-1-5225-2021-4.ch006

García-Sánchez, S., & Hernández-Guerra, C. (2017). Academic ESP Oral Production: Moving Forward Towards Local and Global Awareness. In L. Leavitt, S. Wisdom, & K. Leavitt (Eds.), *Cultural Awareness and Competency Development in Higher Education* (pp. 255–271). Hershey, PA: IGI Global. doi:10.4018/978-1-5225-2145-7.ch015

Garg, B., Khanna, P., & Khanna, A. (2017). Chronic Mental Illness and the Changing Scope of Intervention Strategies, Diagnosis, and Treatment in Child and Adolescent Population. In B. Prasad (Ed.), *Chronic Mental Illness and the Changing Scope of Intervention Strategies, Diagnosis, and Treatment* (pp. 258–269). Hershey, PA: IGI Global. doi:10.4018/978-1-5225-0519-8.ch014

Ghosh, N., Sinha, V. K., & Poddar, S. (2016). Vocational Rehabilitation: Recent Trends and Issues in Vocational Rehabilitation of People with ID. In R. Gopalan (Ed.), *Handbook of Research on Diagnosing, Treating, and Managing Intellectual Disabilities* (pp. 310–330). Hershey, PA: IGI Global. doi:10.4018/978-1-5225-0089-6.ch016

Giannouli, V. (2016). Crime and Legal Issues among Intellectually Disabled Individuals. In R. Gopalan (Ed.), *Handbook of Research on Diagnosing, Treating, and Managing Intellectual Disabilities* (pp. 346–369). Hershey, PA: IGI Global. doi:10.4018/978-1-5225-0089-6.ch018

Gibbon, M., Duffy, C. M., Taylor, G., & Laniel, S. (2016). Juvenile Idiopathic Arthritis (JIA) and Education in Primary School Children. In M. Gordon (Ed.), *Challenges Surrounding the Education of Children with Chronic Diseases* (pp. 59–84). Hershey, PA: IGI Global. doi:10.4018/978-1-4666-9452-1.ch004

Gibbon, T. C., Cline, J., Schwilk, C. L., Hosfelt, P. D., & Bateman, D. F. (2016). The Educational Rights of Students with Chronic Disease. In M. Gordon (Ed.), *Challenges Surrounding the Education of Children with Chronic Diseases* (pp. 199–226). Hershey, PA: IGI Global. doi:10.4018/978-1-4666-9452-1.ch010

Gibbon, T. C., Schwilk, C. L., Cline, J., Matthews, K., Sweigart, K., Ferguson, E., & Bateman, D. F. (2016). Case Studies of Chronically Ill Children: Implications for Education Professionals. In M. Gordon (Ed.), *Challenges Surrounding the Education of Children with Chronic Diseases* (pp. 263–296). Hershey, PA: IGI Global. doi:10.4018/978-1-4666-9452-1.ch013

Gopal, A. (2016). Academic Experiences of International Graduate Students: The Canadian Perspective in the Context of Internationalization. In K. Bista & C. Foster (Eds.), *Exploring the Social and Academic Experiences of International Students in Higher Education Institutions* (pp. 21–37). Hershey, PA: IGI Global. doi:10.4018/978-1-4666-9749-2.ch002

Gopalan, R. T. (2016). Intellectual Disability: From History to Recent Trends. In R. Gopalan (Ed.), *Handbook of Research on Diagnosing, Treating, and Managing Intellectual Disabilities* (pp. 1–10). Hershey, PA: IGI Global. doi:10.4018/978-1-5225-0089-6.ch001

Gopalan, R. T., & Agustus, P. (2016). Sexuality, Parenting Skills, and Related Issues in Persons with Intellectual Disability. In R. Gopalan (Ed.), *Handbook of Research on Diagnosing, Treating, and Managing Intellectual Disabilities* (pp. 386–395). Hershey, PA: IGI Global. doi:10.4018/978-1-5225-0089-6.ch020

Gordon, M. (2016). Parents as Advocates for Children with IBD at School. In M. Gordon (Ed.), *Challenges Surrounding the Education of Children with Chronic Diseases* (pp. 138–150). Hershey, PA: IGI Global. doi:10.4018/978-1-4666-9452-1.ch007

Gordon, M. (2016). The School Experiences of Children with Inflammatory Bowel Disease. In M. Gordon (Ed.), *Challenges Surrounding the Education of Children with Chronic Diseases* (pp. 1–11). Hershey, PA: IGI Global. doi:10.4018/978-1-4666-9452-1.ch001

Graham, D., Killoran, I., & Parekh, G. (2016). Supporting Students' Mental Health and Emotional Well-Being in Inclusive Classrooms. In M. Gordon (Ed.), *Challenges Surrounding the Education of Children with Chronic Diseases* (pp. 86–116). Hershey, PA: IGI Global. doi:10.4018/978-1-4666-9452-1.ch005

Green, W. M., & De Cruz, V. (2017). Enhancing Intercultural Competency Though Co-Curricular Activities in Higher Education: Three Examples From an American University. In A. Shahriar & G. Syed (Eds.), *Student Culture and Identity in Higher Education* (pp. 59–74). Hershey, PA: IGI Global. doi:10.4018/978-1-5225-2551-6.ch004

Gupta, S. K. (2016). Use of Assistive Technology to Empower Persons with Intellectual Disabilities. In R. Gopalan (Ed.), *Handbook of Research on Diagnosing, Treating, and Managing Intellectual Disabilities* (pp. 331–345). Hershey, PA: IGI Global. doi:10.4018/978-1-5225-0089-6.ch017

Halder, S., & Mahato, A. (2017). Cognitive Remediation Therapy in Chronic Schizophrenia. In B. Prasad (Ed.), *Chronic Mental Illness and the Changing Scope of Intervention Strategies, Diagnosis, and Treatment* (pp. 292–307). Hershey, PA: IGI Global. doi:10.4018/978-1-5225-0519-8.ch016

Hansson, T. (2015). Modeling and Analyzing Contextual Influences. In T. Hansson (Ed.), *Contemporary Approaches to Activity Theory: Interdisciplinary Perspectives on Human Behavior* (pp. 249–263). Hershey, PA: IGI Global. doi:10.4018/978-1-4666-6603-0.ch015

Hart, A., Lantz, C., & Montague, J. (2017). Identity, Power, and Discomfort: Developing Intercultural Competence Through Transformative Learning. In A. Shahriar & G. Syed (Eds.), *Student Culture and Identity in Higher Education* (pp. 38–58). Hershey, PA: IGI Global. doi:10.4018/978-1-5225-2551-6.ch003

Hashim, A. H., Kaur, M., Bahar, N., & Ismail, W. S. (2016). Mental Health Issues among Family Members of Children with Mental Disability. In R. Gopalan (Ed.), *Handbook of Research on Diagnosing, Treating, and Managing Intellectual Disabilities* (pp. 54–81). Hershey, PA: IGI Global. doi:10.4018/978-1-5225-0089-6.ch004

Hazarika, M., & Choudhury, S. (2016). Attitude towards People with Intellectual Disabilities (PWID). In R. Gopalan (Ed.), *Handbook of Research on Diagnosing, Treating, and Managing Intellectual Disabilities* (pp. 237–261). Hershey, PA: IGI Global. doi:10.4018/978-1-5225-0089-6.ch013

Hennessy, J. L., Smythe, L., Abbott, M., & Hughes, F. A. (2017). Mental Health Support Workers: An Evolving Workforce. In M. Smith & A. Jury (Eds.), *Workforce Development Theory and Practice in the Mental Health Sector* (pp. 200–221). Hershey, PA: IGI Global. doi:10.4018/978-1-5225-1874-7.ch010

Hill, C. W., & Withy, K. (2017). Rural Mental Health Workforce Development in Hawai'i and the US-Affiliated Pacific Islands. In M. Smith & A. Jury (Eds.), *Workforce Development Theory and Practice in the Mental Health Sector* (pp. 60–89). Hershey, PA: IGI Global. doi:10.4018/978-1-5225-1874-7.ch003

Hoffman, J. C., & Osipoff, J. N. (2016). Type 1 Diabetes Mellitus in the Inclusive School Setting: Daily and Long Term Effects on Education. In M. Gordon (Ed.), *Challenges Surrounding the Education of Children with Chronic Diseases* (pp. 26–58). Hershey, PA: IGI Global. doi:10.4018/978-1-4666-9452-1.ch003

Hoge, M. A., Stuart, G. W., Morris, J. A., Huey, L. Y., Flaherty, M. T., & Paris, M. Jr. (2017). Behavioral Health Workforce Development in the United States. In M. Smith & A. Jury (Eds.), *Workforce Development Theory and Practice in the Mental Health Sector* (pp. 37–59). Hershey, PA: IGI Global. doi:10.4018/978-1-5225-1874-7.ch002

Huda, M., Sabani, N., Shahrill, M., Jasmi, K. A., Basiron, B., & Mustari, M. I. (2017). Empowering Learning Culture as Student Identity Construction in Higher Education. In A. Shahriar & G. Syed (Eds.), *Student Culture and Identity in Higher Education* (pp. 160–179). Hershey, PA: IGI Global. doi:10.4018/978-1-5225-2551-6.ch010

Isik, I. (2017). Organizations and Exposure to Trauma at a Collective Level: The Taxonomy of Potentially Traumatic Events. In S. Háša & R. Brunet-Thornton (Eds.), *Impact of Organizational Trauma on Workplace Behavior and Performance* (pp. 18–56). Hershey, PA: IGI Global. doi:10.4018/978-1-5225-2021-4.ch002

Islam, S. M., Tabassum, R., Colet, P. C., Cruz, J. P., Dey, S., Rawal, L. B., & Islam, A. (2017). Human Resources for Mental Health in Low and Middle Income Countries: Evidence from Bangladesh. In M. Smith & A. Jury (Eds.), *Workforce Development Theory and Practice in the Mental Health Sector* (pp. 144–164). Hershey, PA: IGI Global. doi:10.4018/978-1-5225-1874-7.ch007

Janus, M., & Siddiqua, A. (2016). Challenges for Children with Special Health Needs at the Time of Transition to School. In M. Gordon (Ed.), *Challenges Surrounding the Education of Children with Chronic Diseases* (pp. 165–197). Hershey, PA: IGI Global. doi:10.4018/978-1-4666-9452-1.ch009

Jerabek, I., & Muoio, D. (2017). The Stress Profile: The Influence of Personal Characteristics on Response to Occupational Trauma. In S. Háša & R. Brunet-Thornton (Eds.), *Impact of Organizational Trauma on Workplace Behavior and Performance* (pp. 77–119). Hershey, PA: IGI Global. doi:10.4018/978-1-5225-2021-4.ch004

Jha, S., Khanna, A., & Khanna, P. (2017). Advanced Intervention Strategies for Suicide in Patients with Chronic Mental Illness. In B. Prasad (Ed.), *Chronic Mental Illness and the Changing Scope of Intervention Strategies, Diagnosis, and Treatment* (pp. 271–291). Hershey, PA: IGI Global. doi:10.4018/978-1-5225-0519-8.ch015

Jóhannsdóttir, T. (2015). Responsive Practices in Online Teacher Education. In T. Hansson (Ed.), *Contemporary Approaches to Activity Theory: Interdisciplinary Perspectives on Human Behavior* (pp. 1–18). Hershey, PA: IGI Global. doi:10.4018/978-1-4666-6603-0.ch001

Johansson, K. (2015). Collaborative Music Making and Artistic Agency. In T. Hansson (Ed.), *Contemporary Approaches to Activity Theory: Interdisciplinary Perspectives on Human Behavior* (pp. 73–91). Hershey, PA: IGI Global. doi:10.4018/978-1-4666-6603-0.ch005

Jonasson, C. (2015). Vocational Learning Mediated by Constructive Competition. In T. Hansson (Ed.), *Contemporary Approaches to Activity Theory: Interdisciplinary Perspectives on Human Behavior* (pp. 92–107). Hershey, PA: IGI Global. doi:10.4018/978-1-4666-6603-0.ch006

Kakkori, L., & Huttunen, R. (2015). Vygotsky, Heidegger, and Gadamer on Moral Development. In T. Hansson (Ed.), *Contemporary Approaches to Activity Theory: Interdisciplinary Perspectives on Human Behavior* (pp. 323–336). Hershey, PA: IGI Global. doi:10.4018/978-1-4666-6603-0.ch019

Kaushik, P., & Singh, T. B. (2017). Predictors of Expressed Emotion, Caregiver's Burden, and Quality of Life in Chronic Mental Illness. In B. Prasad (Ed.), *Chronic Mental Illness and the Changing Scope of Intervention Strategies, Diagnosis, and Treatment* (pp. 143–163). Hershey, PA: IGI Global. doi:10.4018/978-1-5225-0519-8.ch008

Kennedy, B. F., & McLaughlin, P. M. (2017). Growing Global STEM Learning in Higher Education. In L. Leavitt, S. Wisdom, & K. Leavitt (Eds.), *Cultural Awareness and Competency Development in Higher Education* (pp. 132–147). Hershey, PA: IGI Global. doi:10.4018/978-1-5225-2145-7.ch008

Kılıç, B. (2017). An Organizational Trauma Intervention: A Case From Turkey. In S. Háša & R. Brunet-Thornton (Eds.), *Impact of Organizational Trauma on Workplace Behavior and Performance* (pp. 264–277). Hershey, PA: IGI Global. doi:10.4018/978-1-5225-2021-4.ch011

Kim, Y. K., Carter, J. L., & Armstrong, C. L. (2017). Civic Responsibility Development Among College Students: How Is It Different by Student Race? In L. Leavitt, S. Wisdom, & K. Leavitt (Eds.), *Cultural Awareness and Competency Development in Higher Education* (pp. 92–110). Hershey, PA: IGI Global. doi:10.4018/978-1-5225-2145-7.ch006

Koning, A., & Poole, S. J. (2017). Supporting People Who Experience Co-Existing Mental Health and Addiction Problems: A National Approach to Improving Responsiveness in Aotearoa New Zealand. In M. Smith & A. Jury (Eds.), *Workforce Development Theory and Practice in the Mental Health Sector* (pp. 251–270). Hershey, PA: IGI Global. doi:10.4018/978-1-5225-1874-7.ch012

Kučera, D. (2017). The Potential of Spirituality for the Treatment of Organizational Trauma. In S. Háša & R. Brunet-Thornton (Eds.), *Impact of Organizational Trauma on Workplace Behavior and Performance* (pp. 295–317). Hershey, PA: IGI Global. doi:10.4018/978-1-5225-2021-4.ch013

Kukreti, P., Khanna, P., & Khanna, A. (2017). Chronic Mental Illnesses and Homelessness. In B. Prasad (Ed.), *Chronic Mental Illness and the Changing Scope of Intervention Strategies, Diagnosis, and Treatment* (pp. 1–20). Hershey, PA: IGI Global. doi:10.4018/978-1-5225-0519-8.ch001

Kyhlbäck, H. (2015). Game Construction Activity in Higher Education. In T. Hansson (Ed.), *Contemporary Approaches to Activity Theory: Interdisciplinary Perspectives on Human Behavior* (pp. 54–71). Hershey, PA: IGI Global. doi:10.4018/978-1-4666-6603-0.ch004

Laffier, J., Petrarca, D., & Hughes, J. M. (2017). The Need for Promoting and Developing Cultural Competency in Future Teachers. In L. Leavitt, S. Wisdom, & K. Leavitt (Eds.), *Cultural Awareness and Competency Development in Higher Education* (pp. 148–167). Hershey, PA: IGI Global. doi:10.4018/978-1-5225-2145-7.ch009

Lawson, R., & Dunnachie, B. (2017). Workforce Development in the Child and Adolescent Mental Health Sector: The Challenge of Rolling out a Specialist Eating Disorders Treatment in New Zealand. In M. Smith & A. Jury (Eds.), *Workforce Development Theory and Practice in the Mental Health Sector* (pp. 271–283). Hershey, PA: IGI Global. doi:10.4018/978-1-5225-1874-7.ch013

Lewis, A. (2016). Making Meaning of Race and Racialization in the Lives of Five International Graduate Students. In K. Bista & C. Foster (Eds.), *Exploring the Social and Academic Experiences of International Students in Higher Education Institutions* (pp. 59–78). Hershey, PA: IGI Global. doi:10.4018/978-1-4666-9749-2.ch004

Li, M. (2016). Learning the Rules of the Game: Issues Affecting Academic Acculturation of Asian International Students in New Zealand Universities. In K. Bista & C. Foster (Eds.), *Exploring the Social and Academic Experiences of International Students in Higher Education Institutions* (pp. 38–58). Hershey, PA: IGI Global. doi:10.4018/978-1-4666-9749-2.ch003

Lin, X., & Baker, B. A. (2017). Challenges and Changing Attitudes for Chinese Women Seeking PhDs. In A. Shahriar & G. Syed (Eds.), *Student Culture and Identity in Higher Education* (pp. 76–92). Hershey, PA: IGI Global. doi:10.4018/978-1-5225-2551-6.ch005

Linge, A. (2015). Creative Musical Practice in an Educational Context. In T. Hansson (Ed.), *Contemporary Approaches to Activity Theory: Interdisciplinary Perspectives on Human Behavior* (pp. 143–160). Hershey, PA: IGI Global. doi:10.4018/978-1-4666-6603-0.ch009

M., K., & Boominathan, P. (2016). Assessment and Management of Communication Skills in Individuals with Intellectual Disability: Perspectives in the 21st Century. In R. Gopalan (Ed.), *Handbook of Research on Diagnosing, Treating, and Managing Intellectual Disabilities* (pp. 156-185). Hershey, PA: IGI Global. doi:10.4018/978-1-5225-0089-6.ch009

Mahato, A., & Halder, S. (2017). Disability in Schizophrenia: The Psychosocial and Neurocognitive Perspective. In B. Prasad (Ed.), *Chronic Mental Illness and the Changing Scope of Intervention Strategies, Diagnosis, and Treatment* (pp. 188–202). Hershey, PA: IGI Global. doi:10.4018/978-1-5225-0519-8.ch010

Maich, K., Belcher, C., Sider, S., & Johnson, N. (2016). Using Children's Literature to Support Social-Emotional Growth in the Classroom: A Bibliotherapeutic Approach to Education about Chronic Disease. In M. Gordon (Ed.), *Challenges Surrounding the Education of Children with Chronic Diseases* (pp. 297–322). Hershey, PA: IGI Global. doi:10.4018/978-1-4666-9452-1.ch014

Manguvo, A. (2016). Negotiating the Boundaries of American Blackness: The Experiences of African Students in the United States. In K. Bista & C. Foster (Eds.), *Exploring the Social and Academic Experiences of International Students in Higher Education Institutions* (pp. 79–95). Hershey, PA: IGI Global. doi:10.4018/978-1-4666-9749-2.ch005

Martin, K. J. (2017). International Students in Higher Education: More Than a Fish Out of Water. In L. Leavitt, S. Wisdom, & K. Leavitt (Eds.), *Cultural Awareness and Competency Development in Higher Education* (pp. 21–39). Hershey, PA: IGI Global. doi:10.4018/978-1-5225-2145-7.ch002

McKay, R., Coombs, T., & Anderson, J. M. (2017). Mental Health and Addiction Workforce Development in Australia: Never the Twain to Meet? In M. Smith & A. Jury (Eds.), *Workforce Development Theory and Practice in the Mental Health Sector* (pp. 90–105). Hershey, PA: IGI Global. doi:10.4018/978-1-5225-1874-7.ch004

McMillan, S. J., & Ripley, C. D. (2017). Persistence Profiles and Institutional Initiatives: Helping Students Become Ready for the World. In L. Leavitt, S. Wisdom, & K. Leavitt (Eds.), *Cultural Awareness and Competency Development in Higher Education* (pp. 288–303). Hershey, PA: IGI Global. doi:10.4018/978-1-5225-2145-7.ch017

Mueller, C., King, M. D., & Klar, D. (2017). Reframing White Privilege. In L. Leavitt, S. Wisdom, & K. Leavitt (Eds.), *Cultural Awareness and Competency Development in Higher Education* (pp. 61–74). Hershey, PA: IGI Global. doi:10.4018/978-1-5225-2145-7.ch004

Mugambwa, J., Mwebaza, S., & Namubiru, B. (2017). Gender Equality Policy, Elites and Women Empowerment in Higher Education Institutions. In A. Shahriar & G. Syed (Eds.), *Student Culture and Identity in Higher Education* (pp. 93–110). Hershey, PA: IGI Global. doi:10.4018/978-1-5225-2551-6.ch006

Mwangi, C. A., Peralta, A. M., Fries-Britt, S., & Daoud, N. (2016). Academic Motivation and Experiences of International Students of Color in STEM. In K. Bista & C. Foster (Eds.), *Exploring the Social and Academic Experiences of International Students in Higher Education Institutions* (pp. 197–211). Hershey, PA: IGI Global. doi:10.4018/978-1-4666-9749-2.ch011

Myers, Z. R., Swearer, S. M., Martin, M. J., & Palacios, R. (2017). Cyberbullying and Traditional Bullying: The Experiences of Poly-Victimization Among Diverse Youth. *International Journal of Technoethics, 8*(2), 42–60. doi:10.4018/IJT.2017070104

Nascimento, C. P. (2015). Subject Matter Analysis in Physical Education. In T. Hansson (Ed.), *Contemporary Approaches to Activity Theory: Interdisciplinary Perspectives on Human Behavior* (pp. 229–248). Hershey, PA: IGI Global. doi:10.4018/978-1-4666-6603-0.ch014

Pandey, J. M., & Mishra, P. (2016). Intellectual Disability: An Awareness towards Intervention. In R. Gopalan (Ed.), *Handbook of Research on Diagnosing, Treating, and Managing Intellectual Disabilities* (pp. 220–236). Hershey, PA: IGI Global. doi:10.4018/978-1-5225-0089-6.ch012

Pandey, J. M., Mishra, P., Garg, S., & Mshra, B. P. (2017). Chronic Mental Illness and Dumping Patients: A Concern towards Management. In B. Prasad (Ed.), *Chronic Mental Illness and the Changing Scope of Intervention Strategies, Diagnosis, and Treatment* (pp. 40–57). Hershey, PA: IGI Global. doi:10.4018/978-1-5225-0519-8.ch003

Pena, P. A., Van den Broucke, S., Sylin, M., Leysen, J., & de Soir, E. (2017). Definitions, Typologies, and Processes Involved in Organizational Trauma: A Literature Review. In S. Háša & R. Brunet-Thornton (Eds.), *Impact of Organizational Trauma on Workplace Behavior and Performance* (pp. 1–17). Hershey, PA: IGI Global. doi:10.4018/978-1-5225-2021-4.ch001

Popov, O. (2015). Outdoor Science in Teacher Education. In T. Hansson (Ed.), *Contemporary Approaches to Activity Theory: Interdisciplinary Perspectives on Human Behavior* (pp. 128–142). Hershey, PA: IGI Global. doi:10.4018/978-1-4666-6603-0.ch008

Prusty, B. (2016). The Stress and Adjustment in the Family of Intellectually Disabled Children. In R. Gopalan (Ed.), *Handbook of Research on Diagnosing, Treating, and Managing Intellectual Disabilities* (pp. 82–108). Hershey, PA: IGI Global. doi:10.4018/978-1-5225-0089-6.ch005

Pulotu-Endemann, F. K., & Faleafa, M. (2017). Developing a Culturally Competent Workforce that Meets the Needs of Pacific People Living in New Zealand. In M. Smith & A. Jury (Eds.), *Workforce Development Theory and Practice in the Mental Health Sector* (pp. 165–180). Hershey, PA: IGI Global. doi:10.4018/978-1-5225-1874-7.ch008

R., A., Prasad, B. V., & Kosgi, S. (2017). Psychosocial Intervention Strategies for Patients with Schizophrenia: In Chronic Mental Illness. In B. Prasad (Ed.), *Chronic Mental Illness and the Changing Scope of Intervention Strategies, Diagnosis, and Treatment* (pp. 58-75). Hershey, PA: IGI Global. doi:10.4018/978-1-5225-0519-8.ch004

Raghunandan-Jack, N. (2017). Teacher Preparatory Programs and Culturally Responsive Teaching. In L. Leavitt, S. Wisdom, & K. Leavitt (Eds.), *Cultural Awareness and Competency Development in Higher Education* (pp. 207–222). Hershey, PA: IGI Global. doi:10.4018/978-1-5225-2145-7.ch012

Rell, A. B., Puig, R. A., Roll, F., Valles, V., Espinoza, M., & Duque, A. L. (2017). Addressing Cultural Diversity and Global Competence: The Dual Language Framework. In L. Leavitt, S. Wisdom, & K. Leavitt (Eds.), *Cultural Awareness and Competency Development in Higher Education* (pp. 111–131). Hershey, PA: IGI Global. doi:10.4018/978-1-5225-2145-7.ch007

Ristimäki, P. (2015). Explorative Actions in Search for a New Logic of Business Activity. In T. Hansson (Ed.), *Contemporary Approaches to Activity Theory: Interdisciplinary Perspectives on Human Behavior* (pp. 181–197). Hershey, PA: IGI Global. doi:10.4018/978-1-4666-6603-0.ch011

Ritter, Z. S. (2016). Globalization of Racism: Chinese, Japanese, and Korean International Students' Racial Stereotypes and Experiences with Cross-Racial Interactions. In K. Bista & C. Foster (Eds.), *Exploring the Social and Academic Experiences of International Students in Higher Education Institutions* (pp. 132–155). Hershey, PA: IGI Global. doi:10.4018/978-1-4666-9749-2.ch008

Roche, A. M., & Nicholas, R. S. (2017). Mental Health and Addictions Workforce Development: Past, Present, and Future. In M. Smith & A. Jury (Eds.), *Workforce Development Theory and Practice in the Mental Health Sector* (pp. 1–35). Hershey, PA: IGI Global. doi:10.4018/978-1-5225-1874-7.ch001

Rodda, S. N., Abbott, M. W., Dowling, N. A., & Lubman, D. I. (2017). Workforce Development and E-Competency in Mental Health Services. In M. Smith & A. Jury (Eds.), *Workforce Development Theory and Practice in the Mental Health Sector* (pp. 284–301). Hershey, PA: IGI Global. doi:10.4018/978-1-5225-1874-7.ch014

Ruotsala, R. (2015). Networking around Supervisors in an Industrial Corporation. In T. Hansson (Ed.), *Contemporary Approaches to Activity Theory: Interdisciplinary Perspectives on Human Behavior* (pp. 198–213). Hershey, PA: IGI Global. doi:10.4018/978-1-4666-6603-0.ch012

Sandoval-Lucero, E., White, T. D., Haynes, D. E., Phillips, Q., Brame, J. D., & Sturtevant James, K. A. (2017). Engaging Inclusive Excellence: Creating a College With an Equity Mindset. In L. Leavitt, S. Wisdom, & K. Leavitt (Eds.), *Cultural Awareness and Competency Development in Higher Education* (pp. 40–60). Hershey, PA: IGI Global. doi:10.4018/978-1-5225-2145-7.ch003

Santhosh, K. R. (2016). Stress and Resilience in Parents of Intellectually Disabled Children. In R. Gopalan (Ed.), *Handbook of Research on Diagnosing, Treating, and Managing Intellectual Disabilities* (pp. 109–117). Hershey, PA: IGI Global. doi:10.4018/978-1-5225-0089-6.ch006

Sato, T., & Hodge, S. R. (2016). Asian International Graduate Students' Academic and Social Experiences in American Higher Education. In K. Bista & C. Foster (Eds.), *Exploring the Social and Academic Experiences of International Students in Higher Education Institutions* (pp. 1–20). Hershey, PA: IGI Global. doi:10.4018/978-1-4666-9749-2.ch001

Scupin, R. (2017). The Concept of Culture and Higher Education: An Anthropological Perspective. In L. Leavitt, S. Wisdom, & K. Leavitt (Eds.), *Cultural Awareness and Competency Development in Higher Education* (pp. 1–20). Hershey, PA: IGI Global. doi:10.4018/978-1-5225-2145-7.ch001

Seppänen, L., & Kloetzer, L. (2015). Micro-Analysis of Concepts for Developing Networking in Social Work. In T. Hansson (Ed.), *Contemporary Approaches to Activity Theory: Interdisciplinary Perspectives on Human Behavior* (pp. 162–180). Hershey, PA: IGI Global. doi:10.4018/978-1-4666-6603-0.ch010

Sertyesilisik, B. (2017). Enhancing Global Competency of Future Construction Professionals. In L. Leavitt, S. Wisdom, & K. Leavitt (Eds.), *Cultural Awareness and Competency Development in Higher Education* (pp. 272–287). Hershey, PA: IGI Global. doi:10.4018/978-1-5225-2145-7.ch016

Sharma, R., & Lohan, A. (2016). Psychosocial Interventions for Individuals with Intellectual Disability. In R. Gopalan (Ed.), *Handbook of Research on Diagnosing, Treating, and Managing Intellectual Disabilities* (pp. 262–282). Hershey, PA: IGI Global. doi:10.4018/978-1-5225-0089-6.ch014

Simuth, J. (2017). Psychological Impacts of Downsizing Trauma. In S. Háša & R. Brunet-Thornton (Eds.), *Impact of Organizational Trauma on Workplace Behavior and Performance* (pp. 120–139). Hershey, PA: IGI Global. doi:10.4018/978-1-5225-2021-4.ch005

Sinha, P., Garg, A., Khanna, P., & Khanna, A. (2017). Management of Chronic Mental Illnesses and Substance Use Disorders. In B. Prasad (Ed.), *Chronic Mental Illness and the Changing Scope of Intervention Strategies, Diagnosis, and Treatment* (pp. 101–122). Hershey, PA: IGI Global. doi:10.4018/978-1-5225-0519-8.ch006

Smith, M., & Jury, A. F. (2017). Key Initiatives in New Zealand's Adult Mental Health Workforce Development. In M. Smith & A. Jury (Eds.), *Workforce Development Theory and Practice in the Mental Health Sector* (pp. 106–129). Hershey, PA: IGI Global. doi:10.4018/978-1-5225-1874-7.ch005

Sol, N. (2017). Fostering Intercultural Identity During Study Abroad to Strengthen Intercultural Competence. In L. Leavitt, S. Wisdom, & K. Leavitt (Eds.), *Cultural Awareness and Competency Development in Higher Education* (pp. 325–345). Hershey, PA: IGI Global. doi:10.4018/978-1-5225-2145-7.ch019

Soni, S. C. P., & Ahamed, P. C. (2017). Understanding and Management of Caregivers' Stress and Burden of Person with Obsessive Compulsive Disorder. In B. Prasad (Ed.), *Chronic Mental Illness and the Changing Scope of Intervention Strategies, Diagnosis, and Treatment* (pp. 124–142). Hershey, PA: IGI Global. doi:10.4018/978-1-5225-0519-8.ch007

Soria, K. M., & Lueck, S. M. (2016). High-Impact Educational Practices to Promote International Students' Engagement and Development: Evidence from Large, Public Research Universities. In K. Bista & C. Foster (Eds.), *Exploring the Social and Academic Experiences of International Students in Higher Education Institutions* (pp. 292–308). Hershey, PA: IGI Global. doi:10.4018/978-1-4666-9749-2.ch015

Srivastav, D., & Singh, T. B. (2017). Comorbidity Issues and Treatment in Chronic Mental Illness. In B. Prasad (Ed.), *Chronic Mental Illness and the Changing Scope of Intervention Strategies, Diagnosis, and Treatment* (pp. 77–100). Hershey, PA: IGI Global. doi:10.4018/978-1-5225-0519-8.ch005

St George, L. C., O'Hagan, M., Bradstreet, S., & Burge, M. (2017). The Emerging Field of Peer Support within Mental Health Services. In M. Smith & A. Jury (Eds.), *Workforce Development Theory and Practice in the Mental Health Sector* (pp. 222–250). Hershey, PA: IGI Global. doi:10.4018/978-1-5225-1874-7.ch011

Starr-Glass, D. (2017). Can Higher Education Really Produce Global Citizens?: Self-Identification and Architectures of Mobility. In L. Leavitt, S. Wisdom, & K. Leavitt (Eds.), *Cultural Awareness and Competency Development in Higher Education* (pp. 304–324). Hershey, PA: IGI Global. doi:10.4018/978-1-5225-2145-7.ch018

Szymanski, M., & Schindler, E. (2017). Embracing Organizational Trauma: Positive Effects of Death Experiences on Organizational Culture – Three Short Case Studies. In S. Háša & R. Brunet-Thornton (Eds.), *Impact of Organizational Trauma on Workplace Behavior and Performance* (pp. 247–263). Hershey, PA: IGI Global. doi:10.4018/978-1-5225-2021-4.ch010

Tavaragi, M. S. (2017). Chronic Mental Illness in Prisons: Global Scenario. In B. Prasad (Ed.), *Chronic Mental Illness and the Changing Scope of Intervention Strategies, Diagnosis, and Treatment* (pp. 203–224). Hershey, PA: IGI Global. doi:10.4018/978-1-5225-0519-8.ch011

Tavaragi, M. S., & C., S. (2017). Global Burden of Mental Disorders: Quality of Care and Unmet Needs for Treatment of Chronic Mental Illness. In B. Prasad (Ed.), *Chronic Mental Illness and the Changing Scope of Intervention Strategies, Diagnosis, and Treatment* (pp. 164-186). Hershey, PA: IGI Global. doi:10.4018/978-1-5225-0519-8.ch009

Tekin, A. K. (2016). Parent Involvement in the Education of Children with Chronic Diseases: Working and Sharing for Children. In M. Gordon (Ed.), *Challenges Surrounding the Education of Children with Chronic Diseases* (pp. 151–164). Hershey, PA: IGI Global. doi:10.4018/978-1-4666-9452-1.ch008

Toiviainen, H. (2015). Interventions for Learning at Global Workplaces. In T. Hansson (Ed.), *Contemporary Approaches to Activity Theory: Interdisciplinary Perspectives on Human Behavior* (pp. 214–227). Hershey, PA: IGI Global. doi:10.4018/978-1-4666-6603-0.ch013

Tran, B. (2017). Impact of Organizational Trauma on Workplace Behavior and Performance: Workplace Bullying Due to (In)Competency. In S. Háša, & R. Brunet-Thornton (Eds.), Impact of Organizational Trauma on Workplace Behavior and Performance (pp. 221-245). Hershey, PA: IGI Global. doi:10.4018/978-1-5225-2021-4.ch009

Tripathi, M. A., & Sridevi, G. (2017). Psychotherapeutic Interventions in Emotional and Behavioural Problems with Adolescents. In B. Prasad (Ed.), *Chronic Mental Illness and the Changing Scope of Intervention Strategies, Diagnosis, and Treatment* (pp. 321–333). Hershey, PA: IGI Global. doi:10.4018/978-1-5225-0519-8.ch018

Tseng, M., & Pluta, R. M. (2016). Educating Students with Chronic Illness: How the Old Service Model Fails. In M. Gordon (Ed.), *Challenges Surrounding the Education of Children with Chronic Diseases* (pp. 227–246). Hershey, PA: IGI Global. doi:10.4018/978-1-4666-9452-1.ch011

Vaccaro, A., D'Aloisio, B., Hoyt, T., Chartelain, A., Croft, S. D., & Stevens, B. (2017). Developing Social Justice and Inclusion Competencies Through Semi-Structured Reflection Papers. In L. Leavitt, S. Wisdom, & K. Leavitt (Eds.), *Cultural Awareness and Competency Development in Higher Education* (pp. 75–91). Hershey, PA: IGI Global. doi:10.4018/978-1-5225-2145-7.ch005

Vora, K. S. (2016). Family Members as Caregivers of Individuals with Intellectual Disabilities: Caregiving for Individuals with Intellectual Disabilities. In R. Gopalan (Ed.), *Handbook of Research on Diagnosing, Treating, and Managing Intellectual Disabilities* (pp. 118–138). Hershey, PA: IGI Global. doi:10.4018/978-1-5225-0089-6.ch007

Vorkapić, S. T. (2017). *Measuring the Psychological and Electrophysiological Attributes of Human Personality: Emerging Research and Opportunities* (pp. 1–242). Hershey, PA: IGI Global. doi:10.4018/978-1-5225-2283-6

Watson, A. L. (2017). Developing a Practice of Cultural Awareness in Pre-Service Teachers by Promoting Positive Dialogue Around Diversity. In L. Leavitt, S. Wisdom, & K. Leavitt (Eds.), *Cultural Awareness and Competency Development in Higher Education* (pp. 223–236). Hershey, PA: IGI Global. doi:10.4018/978-1-5225-2145-7.ch013

Watts, L., & Gullberg, B. (2015). Acculturation Processes and Expatriate Behavior. In T. Hansson (Ed.), *Contemporary Approaches to Activity Theory: Interdisciplinary Perspectives on Human Behavior* (pp. 285–303). Hershey, PA: IGI Global. doi:10.4018/978-1-4666-6603-0.ch017

Williams, G. M., & Case, R. E. (2016). When in Rome: Socializing International Teaching Assistants into the US Higher Education Norms. In K. Bista & C. Foster (Eds.), *Exploring the Social and Academic Experiences of International Students in Higher Education Institutions* (pp. 156–174). Hershey, PA: IGI Global. doi:10.4018/978-1-4666-9749-2.ch009

Wilson, K. B., Pitt, J. S., Raheem, M. A., Acklin, C. L., & Wilson, J. M. (2017). Multicultural Counseling Competencies: Why Is It Difficult to Apply What We Know…? In L. Leavitt, S. Wisdom, & K. Leavitt (Eds.), *Cultural Awareness and Competency Development in Higher Education* (pp. 237–254). Hershey, PA: IGI Global. doi:10.4018/978-1-5225-2145-7.ch014

Woodend, J., Nutter, S., Lei, D., & Cairns, S. (2016). Exploring the Experiences of International Students' Partners: Implications for the Post-Secondary Context. In K. Bista & C. Foster (Eds.), *Exploring the Social and Academic Experiences of International Students in Higher Education Institutions* (pp. 96–114). Hershey, PA: IGI Global. doi:10.4018/978-1-4666-9749-2.ch006

Wright, M. F. (2016). School Bullying and Students with Intellectual Disabilities. In R. Gopalan (Ed.), *Handbook of Research on Diagnosing, Treating, and Managing Intellectual Disabilities* (pp. 33–53). Hershey, PA: IGI Global. doi:10.4018/978-1-5225-0089-6.ch003

Yu, X., Isensee, E., & Kappler, B. (2016). Using Data Wisely to Improve International Student Satisfaction: Insights Gained from International Student Barometer. In K. Bista & C. Foster (Eds.), *Exploring the Social and Academic Experiences of International Students in Higher Education Institutions* (pp. 212–232). Hershey, PA: IGI Global. doi:10.4018/978-1-4666-9749-2.ch012

Zhao, J. (2015). Project-Based Instruction in Teaching Chinese as a Foreign Language. In T. Hansson (Ed.), *Contemporary Approaches to Activity Theory: Interdisciplinary Perspectives on Human Behavior* (pp. 108–127). Hershey, PA: IGI Global. doi:10.4018/978-1-4666-6603-0.ch007

Zhao, J., & Ng, D. F. (2016). Understanding Language Experiences of International ESL Students in U.S. Classrooms. In K. Bista & C. Foster (Eds.), *Exploring the Social and Academic Experiences of International Students in Higher Education Institutions* (pp. 175–196). Hershey, PA: IGI Global. doi:10.4018/978-1-4666-9749-2.ch010

Zhou, W., & Austin, S. (2017). Developing Intercultural Awareness Within Teacher Preparation Program. In L. Leavitt, S. Wisdom, & K. Leavitt (Eds.), *Cultural Awareness and Competency Development in Higher Education* (pp. 189–206). Hershey, PA: IGI Global. doi:10.4018/978-1-5225-2145-7.ch011

About the Author

Sapna Nanda is an Associate Professor in Government College of Education, Chandigarh in India. She is M.Sc. (Foods & Nutrition), M.Ed., Ph.D., and has undergone a Certificate Course in Yoga. She possesses 32 years of teaching experience at secondary, senior secondary and higher education levels. She has been supervising 6 Ph.D. scholars with one Ph.D. degree awarded and guided more than 40 Dissertations at Master's Level in the areas of nutrition, health and education. She has co-authored a book on *Intervention Strategies for ADHD* which has been published by an International publisher besides one book on *Education in Contemporary India* by a National Publisher and three edited books on *Human Rights, Quality Concerns in Teacher Education and New Education Policy: Initiatives and Implications.* Her papers have been published in the national journals of repute and has also presented a number of papers in national and international conferences. Also, she has organized several national seminars/conferences/workshops. Her extension activities include giving lectures to NSS volunteers, Anganwadi workers and supervisors of ICDS scheme, parents and community workers in the arena of nutrition, health, hygiene, yoga, maternal, child and adolescent health care. She has been anchoring radio and television programs on nutrition and health on local radio and television channels, Panelist of 'Swacch Bharat Abhiyaan' and 'Beti Parao and Beti Bachao' Series on Chandigarh Doordarshan in India. She is Vice-President, Indian Dietetic Association, Chandigarh Chapter as well as the co-editor of biannual newsletter, Nutrition News "n" Views published by Chandigarh Chapter of Indian Dietetic Association. She is Joint Secretary of the Chandigarh Softball Association. Her other professional affiliations include an elected member of Academic Council, Panjab University, Chandigarh, added member of Faculty of Education, Panjab University, Chandigarh, Member of Board of Studies in the Faculty of Education, Panjab University, Chandigarh and Member, Board of Studies in the Faculty of Education, Chandigarh University, Gharuan, Punjab, India.

Index

A

adolescence 1-5, 12, 22-27, 30-32, 36, 48, 52-53, 66-68, 70, 72-74, 101-102, 106-107, 109, 119-120, 127, 129, 132, 135, 141, 149, 160-161, 163-164, 167
Adolescents 1-6, 8, 10-16, 22-24, 26-29, 35, 43-46, 48, 50-54, 66-86, 90-91, 101-103, 106-112, 118-125, 127-130, 132-133, 136-142, 144-149, 160-168
adults 2-4, 8, 15, 30, 46-48, 54, 67-68, 77, 101, 119, 129, 148, 160-164, 166, 168
age 1-3, 5-6, 8-13, 15, 24, 26-28, 30-32, 34-36, 39-49, 51-52, 54, 72-74, 78-80, 84-85, 103-104, 109, 111, 129, 135-136, 139, 144, 149-150, 161-164, 166
alcohol 6, 12, 23, 73-75, 78-82, 84-86, 108, 120-121, 130, 138, 141, 162-164, 166
and Rights of Adolescents 67, 109
attitudes 72, 122, 127, 133, 136-138, 141, 149, 160, 163-166

B

behaviours 4, 11-12, 23, 75, 164

C

childbirth 24-25, 102-103, 108
coping 118, 120-121, 125, 134, 143, 146-148, 151, 165, 168
Core Life Skills 123-125, 132

D

deaths 4-5, 11-13, 46, 53-54, 72, 74, 78, 80, 84-85, 102-103, 107, 163, 166
development 2, 4-6, 12, 14-15, 23, 27, 32, 34-35, 41, 45, 48, 54, 66, 72-74, 91, 104, 107-111, 119, 121-122, 128-130, 132-135, 137-139, 141, 143, 147, 149-150, 160-161, 164, 166, 168
developmental 4, 15, 30, 49, 67, 70, 73, 109, 123, 130

E

economic 2-3, 14, 31, 46, 53-54, 72, 74, 102, 141, 151, 161, 166
Education 13-14, 16, 24, 28, 31, 39-40, 68, 72, 102, 110-112, 118, 121-124, 127-133, 135-136, 138-142, 144-145, 148-150, 160, 165-166, 168
emotional 1, 3-4, 13, 66, 68-69, 71-73, 75, 120-121, 123, 127, 133-134, 140, 142, 145-149, 161-164

F

family 4, 6, 9, 12-13, 15, 54, 72, 76, 79-80, 86, 104-105, 111, 120-121, 129, 140, 150, 162, 168

G

gender 1, 3, 25, 80-81, 83, 127, 135-136, 140, 144, 146, 149, 163-166 growth 3-4, 14, 23-27, 29-37, 40, 45, 47-49, 51-52, 54, 71, 109, 121, 141, 143, 161-162, 164

H

Health 1-9, 11-16, 22-24, 26-28, 38, 46-48, 52-54, 66-67, 71-75, 77-80, 84-87, 91, 101-105, 107-112, 118, 120-122, 124-125, 128, 131, 133-136, 139, 141-145, 147, 149-150, 160-161, 163-168
Health management 118, 160
healthy 3-5, 12-16, 23, 29, 51, 53-54, 84, 86, 101, 118, 121-123, 132-133, 135-136, 140-143, 150, 160, 162, 165-166, 168

I

interpersonal 84, 118, 120, 122, 128, 131, 134, 141, 143, 147, 149, 160, 164-165, 168

L

Life Skill Education 16, 118, 121, 123, 128, 130-133, 135-136, 140-142, 144, 148-149
Life Skills 15, 84, 112, 121-125, 127-135, 138, 141-151, 160, 164-165

M

Malnutrition 7-9, 23-25, 35, 37-38, 46, 118
mental 1, 4-5, 11-13, 15, 23-24, 67-68, 73-78, 86-87, 90, 108, 110, 121-124, 128, 135, 141-145, 147, 163, 167
Morbidity and Mortality 4, 24, 46, 86

N

national 2-3, 6-7, 12-13, 15, 25-27, 30-31, 43-44, 54, 70, 78-81, 83-84, 90, 103-105, 111, 131, 149-150, 166

P

physical 1-4, 6, 11, 13-15, 22, 24-25, 30, 33, 39, 49, 52-54, 71-74, 84, 110, 119, 123, 127-128, 132, 139-140, 143, 161-164, 166
Policy 2-3, 23, 46, 53, 91
population 2-8, 10-11, 13-14, 16, 23-26, 28, 38, 43-50, 67, 73-81, 83-86, 101, 103-104, 106, 109-110, 127, 136, 140, 163, 166
pregnancy 12-15, 24-25, 27, 71-73, 101-104, 107-109, 112, 122
psycho-social 2, 11, 66-69, 73-74, 76, 78, 86, 90, 118, 125, 127-129, 133-134, 141
puberty 2-3, 24, 27, 42, 71
Public health 4-5, 13-14, 23, 46-47, 73, 102, 104, 166

R

relationships 3, 84, 90, 122, 125, 136, 139, 141, 145, 148-149, 160-161, 164, 166, 168
reproductive 6, 12, 14-15, 25, 32, 54, 72, 86, 101, 109-112, 118, 139, 150, 162-163, 165, 167

S

school 4, 9, 12, 44, 47, 50-51, 74-77, 79-80, 82-83, 103, 112, 119-120, 127-131, 138-142, 144, 147, 149-150, 163, 165
social 1-4, 12-15, 24, 53-54, 67-69, 71-77, 80, 90, 102-104, 110, 112, 118-125, 127-129, 134, 136-138, 141-143, 145-149, 161-162, 164, 166
stress 3-4, 23, 66, 68, 71-73, 76-77, 120, 125, 128, 134, 143-147, 160, 164, 166

T

Teenage pregnancy 72-73, 104, 122

U

UNICEF 2, 31, 52, 103, 107, 120-122, 149, 164

Y

youth 2-4, 11, 14, 54, 66, 72, 74, 79-81, 106, 111, 118, 120, 130-131, 135, 137, 140, 142, 151

www.ingramcontent.com/pod-product-compliance
Lightning Source LLC
LaVergne TN
LVHW081322300926
849161LV00008B/1849
9781522573845